Wendy Murphy's
Law:

*Anything That Can Go Wrong Can Be
Made Right*

Wendy Murphy's
Law:

Anything That Can Go Wrong Can Be Made Right

Wendy Murphy

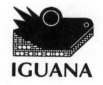

IGUANA

Published by Iguana Books
720 Bathurst Street, Suite 303
Toronto, ON M5S 2R4

Publisher: Meghan Behse
Editor: Christopher Cameron
Front cover photograph: Caroline Acton
Front cover design: Daniella Postavsky

ISBN 978-1-77180-346-5 (paperback)
ISBN 978-1-77180-347-2 (epub)
ISBN 978-1-77180-348-9 (Kindle)

This is an original print edition of *Wendy Murphy's Law: Anything That
Can Go Wrong Can Be Made Right*.

I dedicate this book to my late father, J. Gerald Murphy, for all that he brought to my life.

Contents

Preface

I decided to embrace the challenge of writing this memoir for two reasons. The first was to find a true appreciation for the path I set out on, which has brought me to where I am today. We often get so caught up in our day-to-day life that we neglect to offer ourselves adequate time to reflect. It is our past that contributes to who we are, and it is in our reflection that we are better able to accept our current realities and adjust to them accordingly.

The second reason was to offer the challenges I have faced as an example to my readers of what the human spirit is capable of achieving once put to the test. And how never losing sight of the positive aspects of your life can make all the difference.

We are sometimes faced with hardships that can be overcome *only when we choose not to be defeated*. While many might see my challenges as extreme, it is in how we perceive what we are up against that determines how well we will handle it. I hope my story will inspire others to look for the promising side to every situation in life, while not discounting the lessons that can be learned through the simplest of experiences.

Chapter 1: Regaining Consciousness

I woke in a struggle, gasping for air, choking on some foreign object lodged in my mouth, sticking down my throat. I tried to reach for the object to remove it but I felt my hands being held back. Someone was pressing their body weight against me. I opened my eyes to find my cousin Nancy in her hospital uniform, staring back at me, a look of fear on her face. Where was I? What were those pulsating sounds in the background, and what was I doing lying in an unfamiliar bed? I was feeling groggy, but an overwhelming sense of concern and discomfort was stealing over me.

Nancy composed herself and moved off me onto a chair next to the bed. Finally she was able to speak.

"There's nothing to worry about now, Wendy," she assured me, taking my hand. "You've been through surgery and all looks promising now. I just stopped by because I heard you were awake, but I have to get back to my floor before they miss me. Wendy, it is important that you lie still and not interfere with the machines that are helping you right now. I know your mom and dad will be here soon with more news for you."

Unable to speak, and in pain, I accepted her assurance. She leaned over and kissed my forehead before leaving the room.

Surgery? I thought. What's going on? Nancy was a respiratory technician at the Toronto Western Hospital, so I knew I must be there. But why? Glancing around the room I could see I was not alone. There were a number of beds with people who appeared to be in serious condition, some with bandages covering their heads. All were connected to one or more machines.

What had happened to me?

***

My last recollection was leaving the restaurant in Fort Erie, Ontario. Grania, Don, and I had stopped for a quick bite to eat; a pizza before hitting the road for home. We had spent the long weekend at Sherkston Beach, on the shores of Lake Erie. A large group from our community in Malton, at least forty of us, had camped there. The grounds were lush with green forest surrounding campsites lined in endless rows, all with electrical outlets and barbeques as we enjoyed the weekend.

It was our second trip to Sherkston Beach that summer. The beaches were pristine, and we enjoyed long hours in the water and waves, which refreshed and cooled us from daytime temperatures that were above 30 degrees. When we were there we usually drove our vehicles right down to the water and parked them directly on the sand, playing the car's stereo to create more of an atmosphere. Songs like Bruce Springsteen's "Dancing in the Dark" and Billy Idol's "Rebel Yell" and "Eyes Without a Face" were heard often.

The locale took me back to my childhood, and our family visits to the east coast. Prince Edward Island was our usual destination, with Cavendish Beach my favourite place to visit. Cavendish was a forty-minute drive from where we would stay; the dirt roads brought a real sense of country to the trip. I recall the hours spent beachside clam digging and shell collecting; nothing was more fulfilling than cooking up the clams we were fortunate enough to dig. I will never forget the bitter taste of the ocean's salt water, how we were all careful not to let the salt water sting our eyes. There was little chance of boredom: we children did our best to prolong the day.

When not swimming or collecting shells, we would all sit down to a packed lunch prepared by my mother, a feast that included a whole chicken, assorted sandwiches, and a combination of salads. My mother's potato and macaroni salads were always in demand.

I was born between my older sister, Kim, and younger brother, Jeff. The three of us children grew up in a modest home with a stay-at-home mom and a hardworking dad. Malton in those days was a predominantly Italian community. We had moved there from Jane and Dundas Street in Toronto, an area known as the Junction, when I was seven years old. Both my parents were from the east coast of Prince Edward Island originally, although they had moved to the big city of Toronto when they were younger, Dad at twenty-six and Mom at nineteen. It was often said I took on my mother's trait of "going after what she wanted" in life. I was always searching for new ways to challenge myself, and this took on many forms. I was relatively studious the latter part of high school, taking a more serious approach with time and money spent on math tutors. There was little I wouldn't try if it meant putting my abilities to the test, and that usually took on the form of physical activity. I ran three stairs at a time when getting around our two-storey home. I took little time to sit around and contemplate life; I was too busy living it.

While I was the middle child, I did not go through what most of us are said to experience – the middle child syndrome. I was independent by nature and confident in my overall abilities. I did not feel in any way neglected as a child although at times I lived more in the silent shadows of my two siblings. I believe it was my confidence that sustained me, never really paying mind to any extra attention Kim or Jeff might have received. I was quite responsible and often put others before myself.

It was also a time of transition in my life, and weekends like the one at Sherkston Beach reinforced the independence I was feeling. Putting off a post-secondary school education, I had taken a position with Domtar Construction, in the accounting department. After a recent promotion, I was feeling the world was my oyster. Taking on the full-time position with Domtar offered me more financial freedom. Not long after joining the company, I approached my parents wanting to contribute financially to the household each month, after all, my father had purchased a Ford Mustang for both my sister Kim and me, and insurance coverage would be an added financial burden. I knew the money would help cover the costs, and while my parents were initially hesitant, I was able to persuade them to accept my offer.

Things were looking up as far as my life was concerned. I believed that nothing limited my full potential. I had recently ended a long-term relationship, and friends and extracurricular activities now took up much of my time. Competitive dance was a real passion, both tap and jazz, which was my stronger talent. There was a competitiveness within my soul; everything from gymnastics and cheerleading squad through high school to competitive dance and piano after I graduated.

Since this was our second weekend visiting the campground, we were better supplied with food and cooking necessities than we had been the first trip there. We brought coolers packed with food we preferred, easy to prepare while living in the woods. We were all now at an age that had us doing things outside of our parents' authority. Choices we made now were up for discussion, no longer made strictly by Mom and Dad.

The weekend proved to be adventurous; beach by day, campsites and bonfires by night. Music echoed throughout the park from the car stereos, with as many as eighty to a hundred people attending the outdoor events. Trying to comply with the rules and boundaries of the campground, we did our best to keep the music tolerable. Beer and alcohol were available and added to the festivities. We were all there for fun and to meet new people, and while I knew some of the crowd, there were still several I had yet to meet. We would all usually jump campsite to campsite, taking in all there was to offer before moving on.

While Fort Erie is on the Canadian side of the border, many Americans joined us on our side for the Labour Day long weekend. It was still summer after all, and there was no better way or place to enjoy the hot summer days than at a beach like Sherkston.

***

In my hospital room, the machines hummed and clicked.

Now that Nancy was gone I began to feel very uncomfortable. The machines seemed to become louder. My breaths were shallow, and with each one I took I could feel a sharp pain down my left side.

The tube down my throat made breathing difficult, swallowing almost impossible. There was little I could do to move myself in the bed in an attempt to make myself more comfortable. The pain became unbearable. My legs were raised on pillows while my body was leaning to one side, with more pillows propped behind my back. This offered better support than lying flat in the bed would have, but it was still far from relaxing.

Trying to make sense of all that was happening, my thoughts continued to drift back to the weekend. There were a million questions running through my mind. I now knew where I must be, but not why. Where were all those friends that I had shared such a great weekend with? Where was Grania, my best friend, who had climbed into the van with me at the restaurant in Fort Erie? Where was Don, the owner and driver of the van? Grania sat in the front seat while I moved to the back to lie down on a mattress that Don had set up as a bed. More importantly – why could I not feel anything below the chest down? Why could I not move my legs?

Seemingly out of nowhere, a female figure was standing beside my bed. A nurse. I turned to her in the hope of an explanation. Feeling weak and very groggy, questions went around and around in my head.

Where am I? What's happened to me? Where are Grania and Don? Before I could think of any more there was a slight poke to my right arm and I drifted back to sleep.

I woke, this time, to a loudspeaker paging a doctor to the emergency room. I could feel that the breathing apparatus had been removed from my mouth, and I saw I had been moved to a private room. I was feeling more comfortable with my breathing and swallowing, although the pain I felt down my left side remained intense. It limited my breathing and restricted any movement of my arms, or body in general. The numbness in my lower extremities remained the same. When I tried to sit up, the pain prohibited me from moving much at all. I glanced around to see if anything looked close to familiar, but there was nothing. The room appeared sterile and cold. Not long after I woke up, a nurse entered the room.

"Good morning, Wendy," she said, full of energy – like a new day was beginning and she was ready to face it.

"Good morning," I replied, groggy and somewhat dazed.

"I'm Karen," she said with a smile. "You've had a lot of people worried about you for some time. I know they'll be glad to see that you're more alert and responsive.

Just as she finished her sentence, my father and mother entered the room, looking cautious and concerned. All those questions started filtering through my mind again. What had happened to bring me to the hospital? What had put me in such a questionable state, lying in a hospital bed in pain? More importantly, where were Grania and Don?

"Mom … Dad, what's happened?" I cried out.

My father was the first to speak, which didn't surprise me. He had more of a judicious approach when faced with serious issues, and there was no doubt such ability was needed now.

"There's been an accident, Wendy," he said, with his concern obvious by the look on his face. "You've been here in the hospital for almost two weeks."

"Two weeks! That can't be. What … well, what happened! Why can't I remember anything?" My mind was racing with more questions.

"Wendy, the van you were all driving in left the road at a high speed. Don apparently did his best to bring it back onto the highway but it was going so fast we believe it must have rolled four or five times before it stopped.

"But Grania!" I yelled. "What about Grania and Don?"

I immediately knew something was very wrong. My mother's eyes welled with tears and she took my hand, as my father continued.

"Don is fine, Wendy. But Grania … well, Grania didn't make it dear."

The room began to spin and my breaths became shallower. The pain down my left side was intense and my mind began to race. What did he mean she didn't make it?! How could that be? It felt like just yesterday we were spending long sunny days on the beach, days filled with fun and adventure. This just could not be happening!

I had known Grania for many years, but we grew to be best friends in the later years of high school. She was a real joker at times but could always show the more serious side to her nature when need be. We were glued at the hip. Many would comment on the bond we shared: where I went, Grania went, and vice versa. It was a predictable scene and amusing to the rest of our group. Her ability to listen was one of her strongest assets, and I often turned to her for support. There was something special that we shared, a certain comfort that I had never felt with anyone else. In good times or bad, it was Grania I turned to. She could be my strength, supporting me in times of weakness. We did have a break from our friendship once, for a short period of time, which only confirmed how special the friendship really was.

While Grania was somewhat small in stature, she was great in character. Her hair was her signature trademark, which she wore long with a natural wave. Her eyes were blue, and emphasizing her one-of-a kind character was a brown birthmark right inside the eye.

Suddenly I felt pulled into an unbelievable reality.

My father pointed out that we had all neglected to fasten our seat belts when starting the long drive home; a law enacted but not yet strictly enforced in Ontario. At that moment, I started to question all that we did and did not do. Suddenly *my* fate became a question.

"Dad, Mom my legs, they are numb. I've been doing my best to move them but I can't. Have they used some type of anesthetic to keep me comfortable?"

The expressions on their faces were sobering. I immediately knew something was seriously wrong, a more permanent diagnosis.

"At this point we'll have to leave your fate up to time," my mother began. "Witnesses reported you were also thrown from the vehicle. The side door released from the hinges, and you were ejected. You landed on your back. Honey, there's been damage to your spinal cord."

She went on to explain that the reconstructive surgery had taken ten hours to complete. There were two vertebrae crushed at levels T9 and L1 of the spine, and my left pelvic bone and rib had been used to replace the vertebrae. This was what was causing the pain down my left side. The procedure had been very meticulous, with doctors attempting to remove any bone fragments lodged in the spine while keeping intact any nerves of the spinal cord that were not affected. Given the loss of sensation and movement, it was apparent there was spinal cord damage. The question was, how bad was the damage, and would it be permanent?

It was apparent both my mom and dad felt helpless. What could they say to ease the grief I was feeling? I was on a different level of relating to them both at this time. Working full time now, I had taken on a much more mature position within the family dynamic, within life in general. I was no longer their little girl and this was never more apparent than now. Given the loss of Grania and the many emotions that came with that, my paralysis was not my main concern; anger, guilt, a tremendous sense of loss suddenly consumed me.

If only we had worn seat belts, things might be different, I thought. If only we had been safer in our choices, more responsible, we'd be in a much better place. We had shared years as friends and those times would never be repeated. Perhaps taking an alternative route home would have been a wiser decision avoiding the accident all together, I thought. Then my thoughts went to Don. How was he? What had gone wrong to put us all in such dire circumstances? Back to Grania: had I told her just how much our friendship meant to me? Had I showed the love, respect, and appreciation she deserved as my closest friend? My mind raced back and forth between Grania and Don while the pain seemed to increase with the adrenaline pumping through my veins. I could only think of all the times we spent together, enjoying each other, confiding in each other. How was I going to get through any of this without her?

While I was still pondering my fate, a doctor came in and greeted us with a cordial hello. I was still crying as he introduced himself.

"Good morning, Wendy. My name is Dr. Wright. You've been through quite an ordeal. Are you aware of the trauma your body's been through, all that you're facing regarding the accident you were involved in? Do you understand the full implications of what has happened here?"

I made an effort to pull myself together. I wanted information.

"I know it's not a promising diagnosis, Dr. Wright. Apparently I've received damage to the spinal cord, which has resulted in paralysis?" I asked.

"That is right, Wendy. My colleagues and I worked for quite some time in the operating room, and I'm confident in what we were able to achieve. Your spinal cord suffered compression at two levels of the spine. While we were able to decompress the vertebrae, we're unsure of the extent of the injury. You'll still need surgery on your left tibia, which sustained extensive damage. We'll schedule that for a later date. It'll take time to see how much return you'll have of your motor or sensory skills, if any. It could be weeks, maybe months before we see any real progress. It will depend on what nerves are still intact."

He went on to explain that hours of physiotherapy would be needed in order to discover my potential, with the focus being on my upper body strength. But there would be time to see all that happen. What was most important now was that I get strong, that I gain the strength necessary to prepare for the physiotherapy. There would be a move for rehabilitation, but my strength was important.

"But when will we know more?" I asked. "The pain is quite intense all down my left side. Is this something that will go away? My legs, Doctor, they aren't moving and everything is numb below my chest. Pease tell me this will get better."

There were so many unanswered questions. But did I really want to hear the answers?

"Again, Wendy, I have little certainty to offer now. Will and strength are what you need right now. Healing is a process." And with that he excused himself, assuring me he'd be back.

It was then that my nurse Karen once again entered the room, bringing with her something for pain. What I really needed was something to brace me for the life I was about to face.

"Mom, Dad this can't be happening. Please tell me it's all a dream." All the pain and confusion I felt came welling to the surface. "Tell me time will make this go away and things will once again be as they were. I don't think I could live life any other way right now!"

My parents were able to offer more insight to the accident. They explained it was a vehicle malfunction that had caused the accident and that the highway was also under construction at the time. A family on their way to the airport, headed for England, had been driving behind us and had witnessed the accident and called for help.

Both my mom and dad seemed very grateful I had survived although they were obviously very troubled by the loss of Grania. My sister Kim had been spared any danger, having left Sherkston Beach earlier that day with her girlfriend, Rhonda.

They told me that while Don had survived the accident with very little injury, his emotional state was said to be frail. He was not doing well and many people were worried about him.

Both my mom and dad offered comfort and support for the duration of their visit. However, there were many questions that remained in my mind about where I would find myself both physically and mentally in the long term, including my work.

Having just been promoted in my job, I was looking forward to new responsibilities there. I had joined Domtar as an accounts receivable clerk, managing account reconciliations of the more lucrative clients. The promotion was an unexpected surprise as I had only recently joined the corporation. Michael Levine, the credit manager I reported to, had pointed out that my skills and performance were above average and I showed a keen willingness to work closely with him. It now appeared a leave of absence would be the only option while I transitioned through all of this.

My plans for the Ontario dance competition would be another commitment I would have to put on hold. I had offered endless hours of my free time to the dance troupe, a commitment we all made to perfect our performance.

My mother ensured I was comfortable. She propped my pillows and fetched me a fresh jug of water before she and my father made their way back home. There was a lot to take in. Suddenly my life was no longer a smoothly running machine. I was now faced with Grania's death and a number of questions about my prognosis. My future was no longer full of optimism and ambition, but challenge and uncertainty.

Just how was I going to get through all of this?

Chapter 2: Greeting Visitors

While there was no shortage of people hoping to see me, I was initially apprehensive about accepting visitors. My family felt it would prove beneficial, though, offering me less time to dwell on all that had happened.

My first visitor was a surprise. It was Jim, an acquaintance we had met while camping at Sherkston Beach. We all had taken a liking to him, but Grania felt more of an attraction. She had met him on our first trip to Fort Erie that summer and was hoping to make something of the relationship. He was older and divorced, with two children. Not something her parents would accept off the bat but we both hoped in time, if the relationship did grow into something significant, they would eventually learn to accept it.

Jim entered the room carrying six red roses.

"There's little I can say to make things any better Wendy, and if there was, you know I would say it," he began. There was an emptiness and a real sense of loss in his tone of voice.

"I've gone over it and over it in my head but still can't believe it. It's like a dream I keep waiting to wake up from. How are you doing?" Jim asked.

"I'm much more stable as far as my condition goes," I replied. "I don't know that I'll ever be free of the pain I feel as a result of the loss of Grania. She was my dearest friend, and she would be here to help me through this. Without her now I feel lost, almost frozen in time and wanting to turn back the clock, wishing for an opportunity to redo all that's happened and make it okay again."

"Wendy, while I didn't know Grania long, I'm confident she would want you to go on, to find your strength in healing. I know you were both very close, she shared that with me. She also told me about your resilience and determination. I don't know what else to say, other than that you have a lot to live for – your family, the many friends you have. I'm confident that you can see what you still have going for you. It's by focusing on the positive that you'll see your way through all of this."

I was speechless, although my mind was racing with many replies. What did he mean I had a "lot to live for"? I was paralyzed from the waist down, with no sense of what reality lay ahead for me or my family, during this time in limbo. It would be months of hard work in rehab before I was anywhere near living a normal life, if normal was something I could even hope for now. Before we could say any more, a nurse entered the room and told Jim she had to attend to me, he would have to leave.

What will I face from others as far as all what I am going through? I thought.

"Thanks for coming by to see me, Jim" I said. "And thanks for the pep talk. I'll think about what we discussed."

"I hope you will, Wendy," he quickly responded, before finding his way out of the hospital room.

What was that all about? I thought. I knew then I would have to find strength to carry on as best as I could, an inner strength to take me through all that I would have to face. Medications, physiotherapy, and counselling would all become important factors in getting better both mentally and physically. I would have to move forward with a determined spirit, taking back what had been taken from me. My independence would be regained through fortitude and a willingness to adapt. My dependence, however, presented many challenges, including the simple task of voiding.

I was put on a time schedule, every six hours a nurse would have to use a catheter to empty my bladder. The sensation was very moderate, almost nonexistent. My body no longer felt like my own. With sensation gone and no movement, I felt like Humpty Dumpty, with little balance or real awareness of my lower extremities. The nurse had to take care in all that she did to ensure a less painful experience because of the staples down my side, and it would be some time before they would be ready to be removed. My left leg remained in a cast as it awaited surgery, which did not make things easy when she was trying to move me around in the bed.

Karen seemed a conscientious nurse, always putting the patient first. After facing Jim and his positive perspective on my situation, I tested her for a second opinion.

"Karen, I presume you've been nursing a while now and I wonder what the proper reaction to all that I'm going through should be. I'm mixed with emotions on so many levels and find it hard to accept what's actually happening. I know I am fortunate to have the support of my family, but when I think of the many obstacles I face and my limited chances of seeing a full recovery, there's a part of me that hardly wants to go on. Sometimes I would like nothing more than to close my eyes and never wake up, to call it a day and not feel the overwhelming sense of loss that I simply cannot shake no matter how hard I've tried."

Having Karen there to listen gave me the chance to hear a more objective opinion, and she was forthright with her response.

"Wendy, no one can tell you how you should or should not react to the situation you find yourself in. They are not living your reality. While it's nice that others are compassionate, it's not possible for them to know just what you're feeling, what you're thinking. They might try, but to assume it's a realistic impression would be wrong. They aren't living in your shoes, Wendy."

While her approach was blunt, she made a strong point. In fact, no one could understand the extent of my upset in trying to adapt to all that had occurred. This was something I would have to see through on my own, in my own way.

While Jim's visit was the first, it would not be my last.

The second group of visitors that evening were Christine, Jane, and Matthew Smith. They were a close-knit family that had spent the long weekend up at Sherkston Beach with us and had come to bring good wishes to me. They projected a sense of positive reinforcement in their attempts to help me see a brighter side to the circumstances.

"Hello Wendy," Christine began. She was the oldest of the three – in fact older than us all – with a maturity that brought a calmness to the room. "We've been in touch with your parents and we're pleased to see you're finally ready to see visitors. This is a tragic ending to what began as an innocent weekend away. Know we're here for you as a family, Wendy."

"Thanks, Chris," I responded, with little else to say. "Both my parents told me about the attempts you made to contact them after you heard what had happened. It was very kind of you to show such concern."

Jane added, "If there's anything we can do, Wendy, you know we're all here for you. Everyone is concerned and still trying to get past all that's occurred since our weekend away. Our telephone has not stopped ringing, with people hoping to find out more about your condition and how you've been coping. It's really rocked the community."

"Please tell everyone I am grateful for their thoughts and concerns, and that the reality of it all has hardly set in. I've been instructed to take it one day at a time, which is what I intend to do. The doctors have made it clear that it's hard to fully diagnose my condition, as it might change in the days ahead. They've done what they could as far as surgery goes, and the rest is up to the higher powers that be. Whether I walk again or not, I intend to carry on to the best of my ability."

"I can't imagine what you're feeling," Matthew said. "How a weekend getaway could become such a tragedy just seems so senseless, it has no place in our lives. This has forced us all to reflect on what is truly important."

"I guess this is a learning curve for all of you," I responded. "However, it's my reality."

I realized that there was no way any of them could truly understand all that I was going through, and what I'd eventually be facing confined to a wheelchair: the limitations, challenges, and public judgement on what I could or could not accomplish. Karen was right when she pointed out that no one else could know all my thoughts and fears; they were not living them. While they could try to imagine themselves in my place, they were not there in reality.

"Wendy, we know that you're facing a lot both physically and mentally," Christine said. "You've been spared your life, which is something to be grateful for."

"Grateful!" I blurted out. "What my life appears to hold now is nothing but limitations and huge loss. Are you all aware of the extent of what has happened here? Grania is gone, something I can hardly wrap my head around, let alone accept the physical limitations that appear to be my long-term fate. I want to find a hole deep enough to crawl into and never show my goddam face again!"

Jane and Matthew stood in stunned silence, but Chris spoke quietly.

"I know there's no way to replace Grania for you, Wendy, but I am definitely here as your sounding board. You have all of us to help see you through the rough times and it's time you see us all as your allies. Are you hearing me, Wendy?"

"Chris, I'm grateful for your dedication as a friend but I guess I need some understanding right now. It's a lot to accept, and it will take time before I'm in a position to do that. I'm thankful for your concerns, but I need time with all of this.

"I am overwhelmed with grief and guilt that something more could have been done to avoid all of this. The simple act of wearing our seatbelts would have avoided all of this grief. I ask myself time and again why I wasn't in the front seat so Grania could take the back end of the vehicle. Why didn't I have the foresight to see the dangers in not buckling up for the drive home?"

"Wendy, we can go over this endlessly but it will resolve nothing. The facts are what they are, and your job is to accept what is now, our reality. That is what will allow us all to find some form of healing," Jane said.

"Our reality! What do you mean by 'our reality,' Jane? This is *my* reality! I'm the one lying paralyzed with no best friend here to see me through the trials I will undoubtedly be facing. It's I who will have to face the hardships before me. Grania or no Grania, my reality has changed drastically, forever! I am helpless in my thoughts, and in finding the will to accept any of this."

The visit from my friends offered me some insight as to where others would stand in understanding all that I had lost – not just Grania, my best friend and confidante, but much of my identity and the Wendy I once was.

It was obvious the whole scenario was difficult for everyone to comprehend, let alone accept. Grania was young, like the rest of us. Death was a very hard concept to understand, and it forced many of us into a reality check: how life can deal you a new hand, and all in a split second; how one day life is stable with a carefree feel to it, taking it all in stride as you make your way through the days, the weeks, the months, and suddenly fate takes a detour; how one decision, one split second, can set life – when one is spared it – on a new path. How family and friends often play a tremendous role in our lives, but regardless of their good intentions, well wishes and optimism, we are never guaranteed much by way of life span, and no one is able to control what actually becomes of our lives.

Not only had Grania passed on and out of my life, but my future and my mobility were now forever limited. And very likely wheelchair bound.

Chapter 3: Meeting Louise

The days passed slowly, with little to celebrate or look forward to aside from my mother's regular visits and those from my friends. My physical mobility was limited to my hospital bed; the telephone and visitors were my only hope of reaching the outside world. All felt very bleak. I now felt defeated with my diagnosis and what the future would, or would not, hold for me. I still had many friends wanting to visit but remained selective about who I would see, and usually unresponsive to anyone's efforts to lift my spirits.

Meeting Louise would change all of that.

Not long after I had finished breakfast one morning, the door to my room opened and in came a young woman, bearing weights in both hands.

"Good morning, Wendy," she said in a very French accent, with a smile strewn across her face.

She walked over to the window and with one strong tug pulled back the drapes. A blinding sun suddenly adorned the room.

"My name is Louise, and I've been assigned as your physiotherapist for the duration of your stay," she said.

I was puzzled by this. "The duration of my stay," what did that mean? How long would I be here, and what would eventually come of all of this? I was hardly looking forward to anything she had to say, and it seemed she sensed my desperation while she continued.

"I've looked over your chart, Wendy, and although the future might appear daunting right now, I promise to see you through it physically. I am sure you have many questions and concerns, but I am hoping together we will accomplish something here."

Her personal support and assurance came at a time I felt discouraged, and I really needed it. Feeling I had nothing to lose, I let her know I was on board.

"Hello Louise, and thanks for the encouragement," I replied. "If you've read my chart, I hope you understand I'm still in a state of mourning right now. I'm dealing with a lot, both physically and mentally, but I'll do what I can to work with you."

"I have worked with many spinal cord injuries," said Louise, "and your case is independent of them all. The spinal cord is a very difficult injury to assess, let alone predict what may or may not return. There are thousands of thread-like nerves involved and the naked eye simply cannot see the extent of damage that has occurred. With time, a better prognosis can be made and I suggest you find patience while we work together to prepare you for a more extensive form of physiotherapy.

"I understand that they are working on placing you at Lyndhurst Hospital, a rehabilitation centre that specializes in spinal cord injuries. There is often a waiting list for a place such as that, so it may take time, but I'm confident they'll find you a bed there when you're ready for more intense physical activity."

She then produced a safety pin and explained her first chore was to test my sensation.

Pulling the covers away from my legs, she began poking me with the pin. She started at my abdomen, just below my chest area, and while the sensation was numb, I could feel *something*. She then moved down to my legs and again the feeling was numb, but I could now feel something. Louise went on to explain that the spinal cord is divided into two sectors, one is sensation and the other is motor.

"This is a good sign, Wendy. It appears there are nerves still intact that are responsible for your sensation. It is still early in your recovery so the feeling should get better. It will take time for the nerves to adjust, but this is a very promising sign."

I was thrilled to hear words of hope and encouragement. While I would have to find patience, having some return of feeling was a welcome development. No one knew what time would bring – maybe I would walk again.

Louise explained that exercise and my mobility would be limited until my back fully healed. It was important that the bone regenerate around the rods used to stabilize my spine, so I was restricted from any real movement until that happened. The encouraging part was that there was hope for my mobility to return.

I was overwhelmed to hear such encouraging words of promise and inspiration. Maybe life would be something more than what had been originally forecast: something more promising!

"What I want you to do now is focus on these weights and your upper body strength," Louise continued. "Your arms are what you will use to get yourself around now, and therefore your upper body strength is paramount. It must be strengthened and maintained. It's important that you concentrate your efforts on that for now. All else will come in time."

With that, she handed me two five-pound weights and I began doing lift repetitions with both hands. If upper body strength is what I needed, upper body strength is what I would concentrate on for now. It would be impossible to adjust to the wheelchair without preparing my upper body for what lay ahead. It was imperative now that my attention be focused where it could be most constructive. I counted in three repetitions of ten lifts before switching arms, repeating the repetitions a number of times. I had to be sure not to strain the staples still clearly embedded down my left side, from the back of my rib cage all the way down to my left pelvic bone.

I worked on the weights, Louise worked on my legs. She did range-of-motion exercises that would help with circulation and ensure my legs remained nimble. Being a dancer, I was quite flexible, and my range was said to be impressive. While there was some pain around the incision, it was tolerable. I knew I had to focus on what I could do now. There was a long road ahead, but with Louise's encouragement, I could see a small light at the end of that very dark tunnel.

While my session with Louise was a little more than an hour, I continued with the weights for most of the day, with numerous repetitions until my arms ached. I knew that my strength would come from my dedication to strengthening my upper body. No one else could help with this but me, a test in self-discipline.

Early one evening my nurse came in to tell me I had a visitor, and his name was Don.

I was initially shocked to hear Don was there to see me. We hadn't spoken together since before the accident. I had yet to hear exactly what had caused the accident, and my emotions were mixed. There was little doubt that none of what had happened was anyone's fault. It was made clear that the axle of the vehicle had malfunctioned, causing us to lose control; however there remained a part of me that felt anger about it all. Why had something so tragic come out of a weekend that represented a celebration of life?

"Hello there, beautiful," he began as he entered my room. He had a solemn look on his face, and his posture indicated his respect for me and for the situation. "I've tried to visit more times than you know. How are you doing?"

I didn't know how to respond, with so much that had happened both emotionally and physically. There was a lot to be shared, but where would I start?

"It's great to see you, and not to worry about the time it's taken for your visit," I responded. "I understand you have had your own healing to deal with. How are you doing?"

"That's a hard question, Wendy. I hardly know where to start. My life has been in a fog these past few weeks with no getting away from the reality of what has taken place. I can tell you I'm deeply sorry for the way things happened, and I'd give my life to change the outcome."

There was a delicate tone to his words that carried a true sense of sincerity and comfort. His remorse was obvious and I assured him things would be okay, although I myself was unaware of how it would all pan out. Recent news from Louise brought me a hope that had been nonexistent just hours earlier, and I addressed the situation as calmly as I could.

"Don, we had no way of predicting what happened. I have no doubt you are feeling regret, but there is no turning back. We have to move forward and time will tell us more about how things will ultimately turn out."

My strength surprised even me. I was stern in my response, and I knew I had to be. There was little that could be done to change the circumstances; perhaps forgiveness would be easier, if forgiveness was the right word. I was clear in my head that peace would come, and somehow, we would all get past this.

It was obvious Don felt a sense of relief from my words.

"This will take time for us all, and I know without Grania this will not be easy on you. I guess it's in celebrating her life that we pay tribute to her," he responded.

I had to agree. There was no way Grania would want any of us grieving her loss. She was a true spirit of life, and that is what made her so special. She saw the positive in all that mattered, all that life had to offer, and she held no regrets in her decisions. She seldom looked back and always took the high road regardless of the outcome. It was her free spirit that brought life to those she touched, and her legacy would live on in our memories. This was what we would all hold dear to our hearts.

"Wendy, you have a lot to see through at this time, and I can only offer my full-fledged support. You know if there's anything I could do I will do it," Don assured me, and his words were sincere.

"I feel I'm in a place of limbo right now," I told him, "although I appreciate your words. There is little anyone can tell me about my diagnosis, and it appears only time will give me a better idea of what health issues lie ahead. I have had some encouragement from the physiotherapist assigned to my case, so I think I will bank my thoughts on her words.

I changed the topic, asking what I badly needed to know. "Putting that aside, what can you tell me about the accident?"

"It's an indelible memory, Wendy. We were only minutes from home, driving along the 403 ramp, when suddenly everything went wrong. My steering wheel took on a life of its own, and the van veered strongly to the left of the on-ramp. I did all I could to control the vehicle but it was hopeless. I did my best to compensate, trying to regain control, when I had to hit the brakes in order to avoid oncoming traffic. It was only seconds before we began rolling and I am thankful for the open field we were able to land in. The outcome might have been a lot worse if other cars had been involved, but there's little doubt things would have turned out much better if we had all been wearing seatbelts, a fact that has been made clear by the police and the hospital; such an easy thing to do with such damning consequences. I don't know what else to say other than I'm genuinely sorry."

It was a relief to have Don finally give a more accurate account of what had actually occurred on that fateful day. I had been living the consequences of something I knew nothing about. I was plagued with questions I had few answers for, and this had only added to my suffering. Now I had a better understanding of the situation. Don was clearly not to blame for the accident, which was something I had been sure of all along. I finally had the assurance I needed, and some of the agonizing questions were answered.

"Thank you for a better understanding of the situation," I said. "I place no blame on you, although this remains a difficult time for me in many ways. Grania was a very significant part of my life, a soulmate of sorts, and I can't see myself fully whole without her. I have been forced to re-examine what is important, and my health takes a priority now."

"Oh I hear you, Wendy," Don replied.

"We all made choices that day, and we are now facing the deadly consequences of those choices. I go over and over things thinking of how we might have done things differently, made more responsible decisions but it gets me no further, it changes nothing and only ends up angering me in what might have been had we put those damn belts on!"

"Wendy, no one has greater regret than I do. I was at the wheel of that vehicle, it was I who could not keep us on the road. I have not slept soundly in weeks and the guilt is so real. I look at you lying here and all I can think of is that I am the reason you are here! At least you *are* here, and that is more than I can say for Grania. It's a reality I live with every day, every minute, every second!"

His grief was obvious and there was little I could say to change the situation, so I opted for a more diplomatic approach.

"I thought we both agreed that there was no one to blame for this. It was an accident. Yes, we all might have chosen to wear seatbelts but we didn't, and we've agreed that Grania would not want us putting blame toward a situation than no one is fully responsible for."

I changed the subject once again. "I've been assigned a physiotherapist, Louise is her name, and she's offered me some very positive insights."

"What do you mean, Wendy? Positive insights?"

I could hear the hope in Don's tone of voice.

"Well, it appears my spinal cord has not been severed, but compressed. My therapist did some testing, with a safety pin of all things, and it seems there is sensation returning to my legs. Although it is not a normal feeling right now, she thinks it's something that will come in time. I've been told to be patient, that spinal cord injuries are very hard to predict as far as how bad the damage actually is. It's said that time is the best thing for healing and what return we can hope for. It's definitely more hope than I've had since this whole nightmare began, and I intend to grasp it."

"Wendy, that's wonderful news! I couldn't be happier for you. I'm so relieved that I was finally able to come in to see you. Not to make light in any way of all you're dealing with, please understand how difficult all of this has been to digest for me. The guilt I feel and the endless regret. This news comes as a great surprise and hope for me also. You just hang in there. Something tells me things will turn around."

"Thanks, Don, I hope you're right."

Before I was able to say any more, a nurse appeared and told Don it was time for my meds and she'd need some time alone with me.

Don said goodbye to me at that point, but promised he'd be back in to see me.

It was great to finally see him, although the meeting brought on a feeling of emptiness. The reality of Grania's death was more prominent after seeing Don. The last time we were together was when we were leaving the beach, and Grania was a part of that exit. How I was going to live through this loss became a big question, and suddenly the "one day at a time" theory shared by the doctors came to mind.

For now, I would *have to* take life "one day at a time."

***

As the days stretched into weeks and months at the Toronto Western Hospital, each day became routine. I was served breakfast no later than 8:15 most mornings, followed by a bed bath or shower. My mobility was limited, with the showers proving to be the most challenging, although strategically performed. I was transferred onto a stretcher that was lined with waterproof foam. This allowed nurses to lather me up and spray me down without my having to sit upright. It was a process we perfected over time. The showers were not frequent, so when I did have one, they were never rushed. In fact, I sometimes found the whole ordeal to be exhausting. While I appreciated the process, it made it difficult for me to visualize myself one day showering independently. That would have to wait until my back had thoroughly fused to the rods inserted in my spine. I could not shake off the helpless feeling the showers would bring on, making it even harder for me to conceptualize my eventual discharge and ability to live my life free of barriers.

My physiotherapy sessions with Louise were after lunch. One hour was dedicated to a variety of exercises, all chosen to maintain flexibility and range in my lower extremities. Weights and breathing exercises were also part of my daily regimen to increase my upper body strength and the wellness of my left lung, which had collapsed at the time of the accident.

There was a lot of time to think, and it was the hours between breakfast and physiotherapy that I found to be the most disturbing. My mind would go back and forth remembering all that I had going for me before the devastation of the accident, and all that had now changed forever. My thoughts turned to despair at times while I tried to come to terms with the new reality of my life.

All that changed one morning, following a visit from Dr. Geisler, who was one of the senior physicians of Lyndhurst Hospital, the rehabilitation facility I had been hoping to go to. He arrived with good news.

"Hello Wendy, I hope you don't mind that I have arrived unannounced."

He was a short man, with a receding hairline and beard. There was a kindness to his presence and reassurance in his words.

"Not at all," I responded. "By all means come in."

He approached me slowly, with a message only he could deliver.

"My name is Dr. Geisler. I am here from Lyndhurst Hospital. I understand you've been through some real challenges in the past two months, Wendy. You've been dealing with some pretty devastating circumstances."

"I have certainly seen better days. What brings you here, Doctor?"

"Well Wendy, I bring good news. A bed has become available at Lyndhurst and we are working on your transfer. It should happen within the next couple of days."

"That's wonderful news, Dr. Geisler. I've been anticipating my move to Lyndhurst for weeks now. I know the doctors here have had nothing but praise for the facilities."

"We do pride ourselves on what we are able to bring to the lives of those faced with sudden paralysis. Our staff are top notch at applying both physical and occupational therapies to the people in our program."

I asked the doctor what I could expect when I got to Lyndhurst.

"You will be assigned to a team of trained specialists that have your best interests at heart. They are all well aware of your case and are now awaiting your arrival."

After a little more chatting, Dr. Geisler left me to ponder what was ahead of me. The moment I had been waiting for had at last arrived – the next step in my recovery. I was finally leaving the hospital and going to a world-class rehabilitation facility.

Chapter 4: Moving to Lyndhurst

As I prepared for my transfer to rehab I reflected on all I had been through, and what still lay ahead. There were many emotions. I knew the move to Lyndhurst Hospital was a necessary step in preparing me for the outside world. I just wasn't sure how ready I was to face it.

All four nurses assigned to my room came to see me before I left. They had become more like friends, given all that they had seen me through. I could see how far I had come in accepting what my life now was, and what would have to be done. I had fulfilled my duties as a full-time patient in the general hospital, and there was little more they could do for me. Moving on to Lyndhurst for further rehabilitation lay ahead of me now. It was up to me to adjust to my new life.

"Wendy, what will we do with ourselves without you here?" were Karen's first words. She had been my primary nurse since my arrival and would now have much more time for other patients.

"I'm sure you will all find lots to do without me and my needs dragging you in and out of this room," I replied. "There's a whole floor of patients that need you, and with me out of your hair, you'll be able focus your attention on them."

"You'll be very much missed, Wendy. Trust me when I say you brought a special something to the job each day, a special quality that I can't quite put my finger on," said Lisa.

Catherine joined in. "Yes, a very special something, for someone dealing with all that you are facing."

"Oh please stop, before you make me wish I wasn't ready to leave these dreaded four walls. God knows I've seen enough of them the weeks I lay here praying to be anywhere else. That opportunity is finally here for me. I'm sure you can all understand that I'm filled with mixed emotions. I'm looking forward to moving ahead with my life, although I'm not fully aware of what's ahead of me at Lyndhurst."

"Look at that, you're not even gone and you've forgotten the golden rule," Karen was quick to respond.

"Golden rule?"

"The 'one day at a time' theory. It's the only way to think in order to keep things real," she replied. "It appears you have found your strength and are ready to take the next step forward in your recovery. One day at a time is what brought you this far, and I am confident it is what will bring you to the next stage, the next step toward living your life post-spinal cord injury."

"Thanks, Karen, I guess you are right. You all saw me live that cardinal rule handed down to me by Dr. Wright himself. Speaking of which, has anyone heard from him this morning?"

Before I was finished my sentence, in walked Dr. Wright with a smile across his face.

"Is my princess ready for her departure?" he asked as he strutted into the room looking prouder than a new father seeing his child. "I can't believe this day has finally arrived for you."

"Oh, come on now," I was quick to respond. "I'm sure you've been looking forward to getting rid of me longer than I've been hoping to leave! Given the demands I've placed on you and these wonderful nurses, I'm sure I won't be missed."

I felt close to them all. I am not sure how many patients could leave a hospital saying they had actually made friends with their health care professionals, but they had all offered me such support. They had all seen me through some of the most difficult times. I came in a young woman full of confusion about what had brought me to such a desperate state, wondering how I would get through such a crisis. I now felt I was in a better place and could now picture myself outside of these four walls, ready to explore all that my new life would offer. I was healthy and ready to learn the basics of living while in a wheelchair. It was time to move forward not only mentally, but physically; my life would be different now, there was no question about that, but just how different? What could Lyndhurst do to prepare me for the life that was ahead of me now?

"It has been a pleasure working with you, Wendy," Dr. Wright added. "Although it was a misfortune that brought us together, I've watched you evolve as you took on this challenge and I'm confident in all that you will achieve as you move on to Lyndhurst. It's a first-class facility for physiotherapy. You should feel very fortunate we were able to reserve you a bed there."

"Of course I'm grateful to have been accepted. I'm looking forward to all that I will learn," I answered.

While I was looking forward to the change, a large part of me did not want to say goodbye to Dr. Wright or the wonderful team of nurses that had been responsible for me, day in and day out, during my stay at Toronto Western Hospital. This place had become like my home, and to say farewell to the people who had become like a second family to me was much more difficult than I had anticipated. What would I do without the pep talks offered by my nurses, not to mention the insights and knowledge shared by Dr. Wright?

***

An off-service ambulance arrived to transport me from Toronto Western Hospital to Lyndhurst. My first breath of fresh air was elating; it had been many weeks since I had felt the warm sunshine on my face, and taking it all in rejuvenated my senses. The scent of the air coming from a small flowerbed outside of the hospital was sweet, and I asked them to pace it slowly as we moved under the blue skies.

"Please take your time putting me into the ambulance. I haven't experienced the sun or fresh air for some time." Lyndhurst was only a fifteen-minute drive from the hospital, but they drove slowly because I didn't yet have my back brace and it was essential to take it easy on my spine.

After we arrived at Lyndhurst, I took a few deep breaths before they wheeled me through the automatic doors. The reception area of the facility was impressive. There was a modern, airy feel to the building, with the bright sun shining in through the skylights and bright colours and greenery throughout the main reception. I could see a large dining room directly in front of the entrance doors and a gymnasium to the far left. There were many patients around, all of them using wheelchairs. They all looked young and seemed to welcome me while I waited for my registration to be completed.

Not long after I had entered the building, my family arrived and we were all ushered to my room. A feeling of excitement and anticipation consumed me. The windows reached almost from floor to ceiling, and the outside grounds were well manicured. Birds sang in the many trees just off to the right, and there were flowerbeds just below the trees.

Lyndhurst offered quite a change from the dreary grey hospital walls that had surrounded me for what had seemed an eternity. I felt a real sense of hope while taking in my new surroundings. Nothing I had been told about the facility had been exaggerated.

"Dr. Wright was so accurate in describing the grounds. I don't think I've seen anything so breathtaking at a hospital," I remarked.

"You're certainly right there," Kim responded, leaning toward the window and taking in more of the view. "The grounds go on for what seems an eternity."

My mother then joined the conversation.

"You couldn't have done better as far as facilities go, Wendy. Everyone at the hospital was right when they said you had nothing to worry about coming here to Lyndhurst."

We kept busy that morning organizing my room and becoming more familiar with the building and the grounds. Lyndhurst sat on spacious grounds full of greenery, with indoor facilities that were equipped with the latest workout equipment, much more up to date than those at Western. This was a world-renowned facility that specialized in spinal cord rehabilitation, and its appearance and features reflected that. Many patients had been flown in from across Canada. The average stay was anywhere from three months to a year, depending on the level of damage to the spinal cord.

It was following our tour of the facility, and upon my return my room that I met my roommate. Angie was a patient from Thunder Bay, Ontario, and would be my roommate for the duration of my stay. She was seventeen years old and had sustained her injury while diving into a lake the night of her high school graduation. She had broken her neck and as a result, was paralyzed from the neck down, with very little use of her hands and no use of her lower extremities at all.

"Hello Wendy, and welcome to the lodge," she said, pointing out the incredible view we shared of the facilities. "I'm sure the grounds have impressed you. I've been here for a little over two weeks and I have nothing but good to say about my stay so far, although I'm still adjusting."

While Angie was sitting in a wheelchair, I could see she was not short. Her legs were long, and she had a medium build. Her hair was dark brown and very thin. Dr. Wright had explained to me that the body goes through shock when the spine is damaged, and one of the side effects is loss of hair. It was obvious Angie's body had suffered from spinal shock. I also noticed her wheelchair was different. It was not like mine, which you push with your arms, but one that moved on battery power and was operated by a switch located on the arm of the chair. It was a necessary alternative given her physical limitations. I would learn her diagnosis was quadriplegia: quad representing four, her arms and legs; my diagnosis was paraplegia, with para representing two, both my legs.

"I've come all the way from Thunder Bay in the hope of receiving some of the most advanced physiotherapy available. I've waited three months for a placement here, and I'm hoping it will prove to be worth the trip," Angie explained.

How brave she is, I thought, to leave her family, her familiar surroundings, and at such a difficult time in her life. Not many would have the courage to take on such a challenge without some form of personal support. Angie had no mother, father, or siblings close by to help ease the strain. She was very forthright in addressing the reality of her situation and all that she had been through in order to reserve a bed at Lyndhurst. She was happy to have finally arrived and seemed positive about what they could do for her.

"I have heard the work they do here is pretty impressive," I replied. "I know I was also fortunate to find a bed here, although my wait was not quite three months. I'll be under Dr. Geisler's care while here. Who is your doctor?"

"Dr. Geisler is also my doctor. This is his wing, which means everyone on this floor is under his care. He apparently started this place with three associates back in the fifties."

"You've done your homework, by the sounds of things. Good to know we're in capable hands," I replied.

My mother and sister were off becoming more acquainted with the facilities while I worked on organizing my room; I expected I would be staying here for at least three months. I would be taking on an intense regimen of physiotherapy, with a qualified physiotherapist assigned specifically to my case. There would be hours of hard work ahead of me, and no confirmed prognosis as to what recovery I could expect in my lower extremities. It would be a waiting game.

Shortly after I met Angie, our family came together once again. My father and brother had toured the workout facilities and pronounced them top notch.

"Wendy, you've got some pretty exceptional equipment to see you along your way here," my brother said. "I've never seen anything like it."

"I've spoken to a couple of physiotherapists here," my father added. "The equipment in the hospital is specially designed for those using wheelchairs. There are no barriers to what you can use. In fact, that's what sets this place apart from the many other rehabilitation centres: it has been fully adapted for wheelchairs. You are being offered some state-of-the-art tools."

"That's great to know, Dad, and the further good news is I've met my roommate. Her name is Angie, and she is here from Thunder Bay. I give her so much credit for taking on the trip here, alone, with no family. That seems an awfully brave thing to do, but I guess it speaks volumes about just how Lyndhurst is viewed by the medical profession, the fact that they would even suggest her coming here."

My family remained at Lyndhurst for much of the day. After taking the full tour of the facilities I was even more grateful for all it offered for my rehabilitation. There was little doubt there would be work ahead of me, but I was now prepared for it. I vowed I would do whatever was necessary to adjust to the outside world. Later that night, I had more time for reflection. I thought about all I had been through, how far I had come, and all the work that still lay ahead. I also thought about Grania. There remained a huge loss, a void that would never be filled. I was pleased to be moving forward in my recovery, but I so missed having her there as my friend. It was at times like this that I would rely on her to coach me through the obstacles, the hard times we often faced. I knew she was with me in spirit, although it was not the same.

There was no denying the challenges I now faced, but I realized I would have to move forward without her. It was an uneasy reality, and not for the first time I wished the clock could be turned back, making things as they once were.

Chapter 5: Introduction to Rehabilitation

I woke very early in a new bed, in my room at Lyndhurst. It was such a relief to know I was finally out of Toronto Western Hospital. Now I was hoping for something more. Everything about my new room was inspiring, from the grand windows to the comforters and curtains. It all shouted spring in pastel yellows with strong orange geometric patterns embroidered across the fabric. Quite a change from what I was used to seeing during my two months in hospital, a much more welcoming reality. I was the first to wake and was greeted by one of the nurses, who brought in the back brace that had been specifically ordered for me and delivered late the evening before.

"Good morning, Wendy, I think you'll be relieved to know your back brace has arrived. Now, this must be worn from now on when sitting to ensure proper support for your back since you've had surgery."

I felt a little displaced, not knowing her name or what role she would play in my care.

"Good morning," I replied. "Are you my nurse for today?"

"Yes, I will be your primary nurse for the duration of your stay, although just one of your nurses today. My name is Pauline, and I will be looking after your care until three o'clock this afternoon. So if there's anything you need, don't hesitate to ask. You'll have to be up and ready for breakfast. They stop serving at nine o'clock, which is when mat class begins."

Get up for breakfast, I thought. I had enjoyed breakfast in bed at the general hospital; in fact my life revolved around the bed. All that I did was from that bed. What was mat class? Was this something I had to attend?

"How will I get up?" I asked.

"That is all part of the process here at Lyndhurst. We are here to help you learn how to be independent. I will help you this morning, but eventually this is something you will master on your own."

On my own, I thought. That seemed impossible right now – in fact at any time. I had not dressed myself since before being admitted to the general hospital. How on earth could I be expected to dress myself now that I was paralyzed?

"Well Pauline, I will do what I can but I'll need your help right now. There's not a lot of time if I have to be downstairs before nine o'clock."

Pauline went into my dresser drawer and pulled out a pair of underpants and socks. She then opened my clothes closet and pulled out leggings and a sweatshirt to complete the outfit. Without hesitating she came over to me and began with the leggings while I pulled the sweatshirt over my head; not long after, she began putting my socks and shoes on.

"You don't waste time," were my initial words. "I don't believe I dressed this fast as an able-bodied person. Thanks for your help, and yes, it's something we will have to work on in the coming days."

After Pauline got my brace on, she began to transfer me into my wheelchair. She had a unique way of doing this. She put both my legs between her legs, and while crouching, she bent over my right shoulder, grabbing onto my track pants. She then lifted me, pivoting me into the wheelchair. I was shocked! She was so small in stature. It was a motion so smooth and deliberate that I hardly felt a thing before finding myself sitting upright in the wheelchair.

Pauline began pushing me in the wheelchair down the hall toward the elevators. She gently pushed the elevator button before sending me on my way.

"Well, you can take it from here, Wendy," she said. "You'll have lots of time to make it to the dining room before breakfast ends. Turn right out of the elevator when you reach the main level and keep to your right until you get to the dining room."

Independence is definitely what Lyndhurst is all about, I thought. A part of me wanted the nurses back from Toronto

Western Hospital; they were much more attentive. The other half of me knew regaining my independence was important in moving forward. That was what my time at Lyndhurst was designed to do. So I made my way down to the dining room and was met by a welcoming surprise. Her name was Carrie, and she managed the dining room.

"Hello there! You must be Wendy, the new patient on 2B," she announced. With the dining room full of patients in wheelchairs, I felt I fit in, although I did not know where to place myself. Carrie took care of that, taking the handles of the wheelchair and pushing me toward a table with an open place.

"Good morning all," I announced as she pushed me in to the empty space. "As Carrie was kind enough to announce, my name is Wendy and I'm a new patient. Looking forward to some workout sessions and whatever else this facility has to offer a newcomer."

I was greeted by the many patients already settled at the rectangular table, which sat a total of six.

"Good morning and welcome, Wendy," was the general reply, and many of them immediately asked which general hospital I was from. I told them I had just arrived from Toronto Western. One by one they began to introduce themselves.

"Hello Wendy, my name is Kelly and I was also at Toronto Western Hospital. A diving accident caused my spinal cord damage. I'm level C4, 5 and quite lucky to be alive given the party going on at the time of my dive. I was at the home of a friend when it all happened. It was probably close to five minutes before anyone actually saw me floating face down, unable to move from my neck down. Two of my friends finally saw there was something wrong and turned me over in the water. What about you, what's brought you to this lovely lodge?"

Like Angie, Kelly was quadriplegic, with little use of her hands and arms and no use of her legs. I was initially shocked at her candid approach in telling me what had happened to her, how she spoke so matter-of-fact about something that had so devastated her life. Their diagnosis made mine feel like a walk in the park, as I could still push my wheelchair, feed myself, brush my hair and teeth, wash my face, and do all those little things we do with our hands and never think twice about it.

Spinal cord injuries are described by the vertebral segments in which they have occurred. There are seven cervical vertebrae, close to the neck; twelve thoracic, behind the rib cage; five lumbar, in the lower back; and five sacral, near the tailbone. They are numbered from the top, and so a short form for the fourth cervical vertebra from the top is C4, for the fifth thoracic, T5, and so forth. Very simply put, the higher up the injury, the more severe the paralysis. Someone with an injury to C5 usually has little or no use of their arms or hands, unless the injury is incomplete.

"I'm sorry to hear you suffered such a life-altering situation. I was in a car accident, a passenger in a van that left the road suddenly. We were coming home from a camping trip in Fort Erie," I replied. Before I could say any more, one of the other patients jumped in.

"Sherkston Beach? I know it well! My name is Garrett and I've been here a little more than three months. In fact, I should be discharged soon. I fell off a rooftop and landed on my back, although my injury was incomplete. I use the wheelchair for distance but I have had a lot of return thanks to my spinal cord being compressed and not severed. I'll walk out of here although might need a brace on one leg and a cane for stability. I'm one of the few lucky ones."

"Hello Wendy, my name is Steve and my injury level is C3, 4, and technically, I should be dead. Somehow, the muscles around my diaphragm have decided not to leave me so my breathing is not impaired. I'm also the result of a MVA, or motor vehicle accident, and I'm far from being a newbie. It's been close to a year here for me. I am waiting on accessible housing before I can be discharged, and there seems to be no place available."

Before anyone else could introduce themselves, Carrie returned to the table with scrambled eggs and sausage for me, and while breakfast was not a habit I often indulged in, Carrie insisted I do what I could to eat.

"Wendy, every morning includes a mat class for paraplegics, which will begin at nine o'clock. It's a half-hour class and prepares you for your full day of physiotherapy. It loosens you up and gets you ready to take on the gymnasium and all the equipment designed to make you stronger. Have you been assigned a physiotherapist yet?"

"No, no I haven't." I was a little overwhelmed at all that I had taken in with just the few minutes spent at the breakfast table. I had no idea what else to expect as the day unfolded. At that point someone else spoke up.

"Hi Wendy, my name is Colin and like you, I am paraplegic. I had a motorcycle accident with my level high at T3, 4, but my injury was complete. I have nothing from the chest down. I'll be going to mat class and can show you around Lyndhurst this morning. They should have a physiotherapist assigned to you sometime this afternoon."

Colin was striking in looks with brown hair and blue eyes. He had a presence that no one could deny, and an upper body many would like to own.

"Nice to meet you Colin, and yes, that would be great if you could show me around this morning."

I ate what I could of the meal brought to me by Carrie before making my way to the gymnasium with Colin. There were a number of thoughts going through my head after those encounters. It was all a lot to take in. I certainly was not alone in my fight for independence following a spinal cord injury and yes, this place was perfect for relating to others in a similar predicament. I realized then I still had a lot to be grateful for, given that I had full use of both my arms and hands and with my injury being incomplete. I could hope for more return to come. The few people I had spoken to were not as lucky as I seemed to be, aside from Garrett and Colin. Retaining the use of our arms still offered us a better chance for independence, the ability to take care of ourselves on many levels.

I suddenly felt lucky, and much better off than I had anticipated while I was in the general hospital. There were still many things I could do independently, and Lyndhurst was the place that would teach me all of that.

We entered the gymnasium together and there were maybe fifteen others attending the class, being instructed by a physiotherapist named Jamie. He was full of spunk as he addressed the class.

"Good morning to you all and so glad you're here to start the morning off right! We will begin with some stretching and work our way down onto the mats. Bring your arms above your head and count down from 10, 9, 8, 7...."

While I joined in on the stretch, I was concerned about getting down on the mats. The brace I wore was restricting and did not allow me to bend forward at all. It sat me upright with no way to lean forward or sideways. It was there to stabilize my body frame while the bone grew around the rods. It was estimated that I would have to wear the brace for at least two months.

Not long after entering the gymnasium I excused myself, telling Colin I would meet up with him later. I made my way back to wing 2B. Each push of the wheelchair was made more difficult by the brace and the hold it seemed to have on my torso. A trip that would take me no time at all without the brace was made much more arduous. I entered my room and was met by Angie, who was on her way into the bathroom. She asked me to follow her in; there was something I could help her with. After entering the bathroom she asked if I could help brush her teeth; our nurse Pauline was busy in another room and she had to be at physiotherapy in fifteen minutes or pay the consequences of losing her appointment.

I was thrilled to be of some help to her. I immediately grabbed her toothbrush and applied the toothpaste. The actual logistics proved awkward. I tried leaning into her but was restricted by the back brace I was forced to wear. Angie's paralysis did not allow her to lean toward me, which would have offered me easier access to her mouth.

Difficulty aside, I was able to get the job done, feeling happy that I could be of some use. My feeling of helplessness lifted and I became much more grateful for all I was able to do. Assisting Angie proved to me there was still plenty I could do independently, and that would increase in time. I would be more capable once the brace was no longer a necessity.

After assisting Angie I made my way into our room and began putting things in order. I had been in such a rush earlier that morning that I had put nothing away. My pajamas lay on the bed and the drawers were still open where my clothing had been taken out. I was starting to tidy up when I heard my name called out, and a young woman entered the room.

"Hello Wendy, my name is Martha and I've been assigned as your physiotherapist. We will have one-on-one time this afternoon down in the physiotherapy room. Do you know where it's located?" she asked.

"Yes, Martha, I took a tour of the facilities with my family yesterday. What time should I be there?"

"I've scheduled you for one o'clock. I'll see you then."

After Martha left, I headed toward the visitors' quarters, located just outside my room. I had asked Colin via telephone to meet me there so we could go down for lunch together. I was looking forward to getting his first-hand opinion of Lyndhurst, and that personal tour he had promised. I was also curious about his injury; what had caused his paralysis, and where things stood as far as his rehabilitation. Not long after finding my way there I saw Colin wheeling down the hall toward me.

"Sorry you weren't able to make it through the full mat class earlier this morning. I guess you'll have to work your way into this place and its routines slowly," he suggested.

"It's this damn brace of mine. I feel so restricted in it that I can hardly move. Is this something you experienced initially?"

"Yes, I remember the discomfort my back brace caused at first, although it seemed to subside with time. My brace looked much different than the one you're wearing, though."

"I'll have to ask Dr. Geisler about that. If there is something that would be more comfortable, I would like to see this one replaced. I had to go through a special fitting for this brace, though, so I doubt it can be. I'd like to see more of the facilities if we have time."

"Have you been assigned a physiotherapist yet? They'll have a much better explanation for you given your overall diagnosis and what you might expect. They'll develop the right workout program to prepare you for discharge time. Maybe it's best we make our way down to lunch."

"Yes, I do have my physiotherapist assigned. Maybe you're right, Martha can give me a tour. I am scheduled to see her this afternoon."

We made our way down to the dining room and were once again met by Carrie, who pointed us over to an empty table for six.

"This should work for us, and the others will be here soon," noted Colin. "Many patients have physiotherapy in the morning, and it's not quite noon."

I suddenly realized that I was shifting into what would become a routine at Lyndhurst. Now that my condition was no longer critical, I would now participate in daily activities that would include extensive physiotherapy and some psychological aid if needed. It was made clear that the services of a clinical psychologist were available to assist me in the transitioning process. I seemed to be progressing well, however, through the support I received from friends and family. I felt I had mastered much of the art of acceptance on my own.

Not long afterward, the cafeteria began to fill. The four vacant places available at our table were taken by Angie, my roommate, followed by Steve, then Garrett, and Kelly.

"Well Wendy, how was mat class and your first morning here at Lyndhurst?" Steve asked.

"It was interesting, but not all that productive. The back brace I have to wear doesn't offer much by way of movement, and I was too restricted to fully take part."

"I can relate to some degree," Angie added. "My halo has restricted my movement in many ways and limits my access to showers right now. It will be at least another month before I can hope to see it removed."

Anyone with a broken back must wear a back brace to stabilize the spine. The brace I was wearing had stabilizing bars down the back of its frame, with reinforcing buckles across the front. It is meant to be worn tight, to offer the ultimate support while sitting upright. The benefit to the brace was that it could be removed when I didn't need the support. Angie, on the other hand, had sustained a neck injury and wore what is called a halo, a crown-like rim that is drilled into the skull with bolt like fixtures. Four bars are then attached, and like a crown, they are attached to a vest that must be worn to stabilize the neck. Not a very comfortable addition to anyone's life, and it can't be removed unless the patient is lying down.

"I still remember the discomfort of wearing the halo," Steve added. "It was six months before I was able to have it removed."

Kelly then added her story to the conversation.

"I had endless problems with my halo, and infections where the bolts were drilled into my scalp. I remember having a number of breakdowns with antibiotic creams and capsules as part of my daily routine. I was certainly happy to see it go. I believe it was a total of four months before the bone fusion took place."

"Wow," I added. "You've all shown such strength in what you've had to endure. You inspire me. I couldn't imagine being so confined, and for such a long period of time."

"They all inspire me," Garrett said. "What I've seen these past few months has given me a much more optimistic look on life. There's so much to be grateful for that I hardly look back on my days before coming here. Sure, I might walk with a brace, but I'm a heck of a lot further ahead than when I came in."

I totally understood where Garrett was coming from. Angie, Kelly, and Steve had all sustained neck injuries with limitations far beyond ours. They were all paralyzed from the neck down, with no full use of their arms or hands. I had a lot to be grateful for: I still had my upper body to use in my day-to-day routines, and to assist others. While I did suffer paralysis to my lower extremities, my personal care would not be as limited and I could learn to adapt. The doctors at the general hospital were confident that, with the proper rehabilitation, I would adjust to living in a wheelchair, taking on my life as though nothing had happened. I would learn to bathe, cook, and eventually drive. While these adjustments would take work, I was now in the best place to learn and eager to move forward.

Not long after we found our places at the table, Carrie served us all some lunch. It was macaroni and cheese and was certainly a welcome alternative to what I had been used to at Toronto Western Hospital. There was a chef appointed to oversee the menu at Lyndhurst, with nutrition a major factor, as we were all there to get stronger. Physiotherapy was our focus and nutritional meals and midday snacks would be part of the process. Apart from the mac and cheese, we were served a glass of milk, salad, and fresh fruit for dessert.

Soon it was one o'clock and I headed over to physiotherapy for my first session with Martha. I entered the physiotherapy room independently. There was no one else there but the two of us.

"Hello Martha, I've finally made it here," were my first words. "I know the weeks I spent in bed at the general hospital depleted much of my upper body frame. I was a dancer, but my once well-groomed physique has since lost its shape."

"As you can see, Wendy, we are surrounded by equipment designed to treat that. We have hand weights that can be signed out from the room if you want to work on your strength outside of your physiotherapy appointments. They become your responsibility once they leave the room. We have the pulleys located over there along the wall. They could really help with your back and bicep muscles. Maybe a combination of both weight options could work for you now. What are your thoughts on things so far?"

"I'm happy to see the options available and I'm in a much better mind frame since my discharge from Toronto Western. My eyes have opened up so much more."

"That's great to hear, Wendy, and the feeling should increase the more we are able to work together, the more you take advantage of the facilities here for you. You've survived extraordinary circumstances, getting thrown from the vehicle you were riding in. You've made it through the hard part. Your time here is to get stronger, both physically and mentally, and that will come the more you apply yourself."

"I'm feeling what is possible now that I am here. The doctors told me the facilities here were top notch but I couldn't really picture it yet. What's more, seeing how much more I might have lost had I broken my neck instead of my back puts me in a whole new mindset. I feel fortunate now, if that makes any sense. Although I do miss my mobility, all that I was once able to do."

"There's no doubt you'll miss the life you once had as an able-bodied young woman, Wendy; that goes without saying. Anyone would empathize with all that you are dealing with. But if you keep an open mind, there is very little that you once did that you can't do again, and these facilities can help you in that transition."

My session with Martha lasted an hour and a half. I worked mainly on the pulleys while I was in the gym, knowing I could take the hand weights back to my room and work more on my upper body strength there. I decided I would benefit more by using both forms of weight training, speeding up my ability to regain the upper body strength that I had lost while bedridden at the general hospital. Martha also did range-of-motion exercises on my legs. This was to ensure the legs remained agile while I went about my day, making transfers to and from the wheelchair much more fluid.

I had made my way back to the 2B wing following my physiotherapy session with Martha, only to be greeted by Angie who was once again in need of assistance. She had her yoga jacket partially on. The right arm she somehow mastered; the left, not so much. Although it did take some work, I was able to assist her by leaning her forward and slipping the left side of the jacket behind her. There was a little struggle, but with my assistance she was able to master the second sleeve as well. She was on her way to Occupational Therapy, a session designed to help with day-to-day living for those who have suffered some form of setback or impairment. Through proper assessment and prescription of equipment, the goal is to assist those back to functional independence.

"Thanks so much, again," Angie said.

"The pleasure was truly all mine," I replied. "Angie, if there's ever something I can help you with, I would hope you won't hesitate to ask."

"That's very kind of you, Wendy. The nurses here are wonderful when they're around to help, but they aren't always close by. So I appreciate your efforts as backup."

After helping Angie out I went into our room, tidying anything that was not in its proper place. It had been quite an eventful day and I was feeling tired from all the activity. I had met some wonderfully strong individuals who had shared with me all that had occurred to bring them to Lyndhurst Hospital. They also shared what the stay had brought to their lives so far. It was an eye-opening experience on many levels. I learned that spinal cord injuries are very complex with the results sometimes more challenging, depending on the level of damage. Gaining insights into the effects generated by spinal cord damage had me feeling very grateful that it was my back that was broken and not my neck. This offered me continued use of my upper body, aiding me in maintaining my independence. I had many things to be grateful for, with family and friends readily supporting me in my transition.

I lay down to nap, thankful for the day I had shared with everyone, feeling privileged to be a full-time patient at a well-established, world-renowned rehabilitation centre. It had been a full day, and there would be many more ahead, en route to establishing a more independent lifestyle.

Chapter 6: First Trip Home

My days at Lyndhurst were full. I was able to adjust to the back brace eventually and did not find it as restricting as it had seemed when I initially began wearing it. The part that went around my body was both leather and spandex, which seemed to stretch over time. It would be weeks into my stay before I found wheeling independently much easier, with my attendance at mat class in the mornings now a more regular routine. Jamie and I had worked out a program that would allow me to join in with the class for specific exercises, and I would work on my own when I found the moves to be too difficult with the brace. Overall, we were able to make it work for me.

I was on my way to the patients' lounge when I noticed a patient who appeared to be struggling with the zipper of his tracksuit jacket.

"Can I help?" I asked.

"It's the damn zipper. It seems to be caught somewhere."

I made my way over to his wheelchair and could see that the fabric to his jacket had gotten stuck in the track of the zipper. A slight tug got it back in working order and I zipped it up all the way for him.

"My name is Wendy, and I'm fairly new here."

"Thanks for your help, Wendy. My name is Jerry and it's been five months for me. What wing are you on and who's your doctor?" he asked.

"Great to meet you, Jerry. I am on wing 2B and my doctor is Geisler."

"Yeah, I've heard some pretty good things about him. I guess we all should be grateful for this place. I know it's said to be the number-one facility in the country for spinal injuries. My mom and dad were excited when they heard that I was accepted as a full-time patient. I'm under Dr. Bernhard's care."

"Was it a diving accident that caused your injury?" I asked, not sure if he would want to talk about it.

"No, actually, it wasn't. I know the majority of quadriplegic patients in here are the result of a diving accident but I'm an original – I was breakdancing when I went over on my neck. Not much of a future for a thirteen year old," he added. "It's been a tough time, but I'm getting through it."

"Wow, Jerry, I had no idea. I'm sorry to hear about your misfortune."

"Hey, we're all living a misfortune in here. I am not sure any one of us is better off than the other, although you were spared your hands. I am sure your reality has been just as difficult to accept as mine at times. We are all here to adjust to the outside world. Paralysis is now an everyday part of our reality."

I was taken aback by his candid response, and at such a young age. There was little doubt the transition he was facing brought him not only strength, but also a form of wisdom. He seemed very mature for his age.

Not long after our conversation I was paged to the nursing station on 2B. When I got back to the ward, I was surprised to find my father there with Dr. Geisler.

"What have we here?" I asked. "What's going on?"

"Well Wendy, I have spoken with Dr. Geisler and we've decided you can come home for the weekend, if you'd like to."

"Home for the weekend, that would be great! That is, if you both feel I am ready to take on such an adventure. How do you think we'll manage?" I asked my father.

I knew that it had been months now since I had been home, and there was nothing I would have liked more than to visit. Accessibility might be an issue: our home was a split-level design with stairs literally everywhere.

"Your mother and I have converted the office in the front of the house into a bedroom for you. We figure we could take it one day at a time. It is Friday, so you could come home with me this evening and we'll see how things go. We could pack enough for the full weekend but you could always return Saturday afternoon if we run into difficulties."

"You're serious, Dad, no joking here?"

"I know how much you have wanted to be home again."

"No joke there," I replied.

"There was no way of making it happen while you were in the general hospital but since coming here, you've been in better health, much stronger, and I believe more ready emotionally for this visit. Dr. Geisler was kind enough to prepare your medications for the days you'll be away. If this is something you'd like to do, we can make it happen."

It all seemed unreal. For weeks all I had thought about was going home, being part of my family again. I just was not expecting it to happen so soon. I was thrilled though, and not about to turn the offer down. I decided to question Dr. Geisler.

"Well, what do you think Doctor, is this something I'm ready for?"

"Wendy, we encourage home visits as soon as they can happen. You are here to prepare for the real world, and what better way to prepare you than to encourage you to experience it. You're fortunate to have such a supportive family to make this trip home possible. My clinical position is, yes, this would be good for you."

"Wonderful then, it's been decided. Dad, I will go back to my room to collect some clothes. If you could help me get my gym bag down it will hurry up the process. Dr. Geisler, thanks for your advice and I hope you will wish me luck on this journey."

I was full of mixed emotions – excitement on the one hand, with an anxious sense of the unknown on the other.

Not long after preparing my bag and collecting my medications, I went to find Angie to let her know I would not be around for the weekend. I knew she often looked for me when she needed help brushing her teeth, holding the telephone when her family called, assisting her with many of the simple things we find ourselves taking for granted. With me gone, she would have to find someone else to help her. The great part was, it was the weekend, and with many of the patients going home, the nurses were more likely to be free and able to assist those in need.

While wheeling toward the automated front doors I heard my name being called out. It was Colin and he seemed shocked to see my father carrying the gym bag. Since it was Friday afternoon, he guessed I was on my way home.

"Hey there my friend, you're not trying to duck out on me are you?"

"Colin, no, of course I'm not sneaking off behind your back. I left word with both Pauline and Angie to let you know I had gone home for the weekend."

Colin was from Orangeville, about ninety kilometres northwest of Toronto, making his commute longer; however, he usually found his way home on weekends. As for me, it had been weeks since my admission and the thought of actually going home really excited me. The months I had been away felt like years, and while access in my home would prove challenging, I was definitely looking forward to the visit.

"I was just joking. This is your first trip home since the accident. I hope it all goes well," he added.

"Thanks, Colin. Any tips before I go?"

"Just don't let it overwhelm you. Things will definitely be different and it's important you know they will improve with time. Try to take it one day at a time, and I am sure things will all go over well."

There is that "one day at a time" rule again, I thought. I had quite a bit of practice following it by now, and if experience was any indication it should work out on my first trip home.

My transfer into the car was challenging. We used what is known as a sliding board, a varnished board approximately two and a half feet long. One end is placed under one hip while you are seated in the wheelchair, with the opposite end placed on the surface you are aiming to transfer onto. You then slide across the board to transport yourself to and from the wheelchair.

I initially felt liberated, finally breaking free from the hospital wards and nursing units I had grown so accustomed to. On the other hand, I felt slightly frightened to be on my own. I had enjoyed the security of medical personnel watching over my care since the accident, and that was more than two months ago now. Not having them with me at home made me leery of what might happen.

My anxieties only grew stronger as we took the on-ramp toward Highway 401, heading west. This was the first automobile ride I had taken since the accident. Every vehicle driving around us was a potential hazard, a lethal weapon that could lose control and interfere with us. I couldn't control my thoughts, which were quickly becoming worries. My last trip in a vehicle on the highway had ended in disaster. I no longer took a car ride for granted. My hands became fists and began to sweat at the palms. How long would this drive take?

I had now learned first-hand of the dangers we all face when getting into an automobile and taking to the highway. Speed, combined with the unfamiliar territories we at times find ourselves in, could have deadly consequences. Even though my father and I were sure to wear our seatbelts, the anxiety consumed me most of the way home. There was little my father could say or do to ease the tensions I was feeling.

"Wendy, I will get off the highway and take the back roads as soon as we are closer to home. I never thought about the traffic before we left, and I think you might be more comfortable on roads with lower speed limits. And they'll be much less crowded."

"It's pretty overwhelming right now, Dad, and I'm not sure that quieter streets will change what I'm feeling. The whole experience has my stomach in knots. I hope you understand."

I was really looking forward to making it home and safely driving into our driveway.

"You've been through an ordeal not many would be able to face, especially with the courage you have shown. Your mother and I are in awe of how you have handled all of this. It is important you see all that you've achieved these past few weeks.

"Really Dad?" I asked.

"You have made the move to Lyndhurst remarkably smoothly. You are up in your wheelchair hours each day, you're working out with Martha daily, and you've overcome the limitations you once faced with that brace of yours. Do you see how far you've actually come, Wendy?"

"I suppose I've never really looked at it that way," I replied. "Dad, I feel so lucky compared to some of the patients there. Some have broken their neck and have little use of their hands or arms. I wake up every morning and give thanks to God for all that I have been spared. While I do struggle at times, that struggle could be so much more difficult, a situation I see clearer now that I am at Lyndhurst. In fact, I'm able to help many of them, with little things they need done, like doing up a zipper."

I told my father about Jerry, the youngest of us all at Lyndhurst, who I had met just that morning. I could not imagine something so traumatic happening while doing something so customary or routine like breakdancing. Being a dancer myself it really made me think that we never know just what fate has in store for us. It put me in a new way of thinking. I knew that there would be obstacles throughout the journey, but I had to face those obstacles, and continue to go on.

We finally arrived, pulled into the driveway of our home and it seemed no time before my mother and sister came out of the house to greet us.

"Well it has finally happened, dear," were my mother's first words. "I know you had no idea we were planning this. We kept it under wraps until we were sure Dr. Geisler would discharge you for the weekend."

"Wait until you see the front room," my sister added. "Dad's office has been transformed into a room fit for a queen. I'm just so happy to finally see you home, Wendy, even if it's only temporary."

"I'm glad to be home. It's been months now, and I believe I'm finally ready to take this plunge."

My dad got out of the car and began taking my bags into the house. The challenge was to get me in there. The front door was reached through a patio that had six stairs up. That would bring me into the front office, with a powder room adjacent to it. Any efforts to reach the kitchen would have me face four stairs down to the lower level, with the living room and side entrance located there.

With the aid of our neighbour, Albert, I was lifted up the patio staircase and bumped up one step through the front door. It all looked different, somehow smaller than I had remembered it. The staircase leading up to the bedrooms was in front of me. My thoughts were scattered as I was wheeled into the front hallway, which was not an easy task due to the broadloom throughout the space. It was an emotional moment. Here I was in my very own home and unable to make it around the way I once had. I was faced with stairs everywhere, having little hope of seeing my bedroom once again, or the recreation room in the basement; there was now a whole house that I no longer had full access to and that thought, that reality, only intensified my anxieties. I was suddenly consumed with a feeling of sadness as my mother tried her best to bring my spirits up.

"Look, Wendy, we even brought your comforter and pillows down to the front room from upstairs."

"Thanks, Mom," I responded, knowing little else to say, and not yet comfortable to share all that was actually going through my mind. I felt helpless in an environment where I was once in full control.

The feelings were difficult to hide. The wheelchair barely made it through the door to the front room they had modified as a bedroom and would not go into the bathroom at all. There was very little I could do to get around independently. The broadloom made pushing myself in my wheelchair close to impossible, and the second level did not offer access to the kitchen for meals. It seemed any efforts to resume my independence would only be dashed by more obstacles. My family home was now an obstacle course that I could no longer master on my own. I felt completely defeated.

I wanted to cry, or to scream. How could my family home have become such a dramatic source of power? The situation had grown into something none of us could control or ignore. My limitations in the real world and the difficulties I would face in my attempts to move forward with my life were becoming more and more obvious. I now appreciated the accessibility advantages and comforts of Lyndhurst Hospital. It was like an oasis designed specifically to facilitate us and our wheelchairs; the world outside of its automatic doors was much less forgiving.

"I don't know what to say to you all," I said, trying not to sound as discouraged as I felt.

"There's nothing to worry about, Wendy. We are all here to help," said my father.

I knew they had done their best to prepare for my visit home, and while fetching my comforter from my bedroom upstairs was an easy gesture to perform, trying now to live in the home seemed impossible without their continuous aid. I could not help but become emotional, and the situation was only made worse by my inability to excuse myself and find somewhere private to release my stress.

"Wendy, what's wrong? We have all worked hard to prepare the room for your visit and are so happy to see you home. What did we miss?" my brother Jeff asked. He must have seen the look on my face. Tears began to fill my eyes.

I knew no one would understand what I was feeling; I hardly did. There was frustration and anger mixed with feelings of confusion. I was a time bomb just waiting to explode, and seeking the opportunity to safely do so! My family were not to blame and I had no one nearby to air my frustrations at, other than them.

It was a very difficult moment and one that I'll never forget. I was living in two worlds. There was Lyndhurst, a place that gave me the freedom of access, with facilities and grounds all adapted for the physically challenged to live independently and barrier free. Then there was the world outside of Lyndhurst. Living in the real world would be filled with challenges and barriers that would only cause frustrations, forcing us all to face the limitations the wheelchair would now bring.

Wiping away my tears, I responded.

"I'm so grateful for all that you've done to make this trip home as comfortable as possible. It's just frustrating that the world will be full of challenges from here on in. The simplest of things now require more effort. I see my whole life as challenging and I'm not sure how prepared I am to live that way. I'm hoping you can try and understand where my feelings are coming from."

"There will be challenges, dear, we don't doubt that," said my mother. "But we hope we can encourage and support you. It's important you focus on all that you are able to do, the positive aspects of your life now. It's all about seeing the glass half full."

"I know, Mom. What do you think has taken me this far in my recovery? I shared with Dad the thankfulness I feel in my heart, and that I realize just how much worse things could be. That doesn't take away from the life I was leading before all of this mayhem took place, and the repercussions I'm feeling as a result. I look at all of you, and all my friends, who are not forced to deal with all that I am. There is a big part of me that wants that life back. I'm still asking myself why any of this had to happen."

"I'm glad you're sharing these feelings, Wendy. We all know this is taking a toll on you. Your future hangs in the balance, and your rehabilitation is a big part of your coming out of all of this successfully. I have faith in your abilities, Wendy, and your willingness to adapt. Look how far you've already come."

My feelings were scattered, with confusion a big part of my emotions. I was glad to be with my family when everything seemed so desperate. Coming home was something I had looked forward to so much, but it emphasized my limitations so much more. On the other hand, there was a lot to be grateful for, and by focusing on all the positive aspects of my situation as my mother had advised, moving forward would be much easier.

Not long afterward, my father suggested I be carried down to the living room and kitchen area, where I could help prepare dinner. My family knew how I loved to help, and putting my culinary abilities to work might make me feel more useful. He called on our neighbour Albert to once again assist in hoisting me down the four stairs dividing our front room from the main level of the house. Albert entered appearing more than happy to help.

"Well what have we here?" he asked. "Will my services be needed for much of the weekend? There will be a charge for all of this."

"Not sure I can afford your prices," was my immediate response.

The move down to the kitchen proved beneficial to everyone. I was able to assist with a stir-fry, and there were dishes to be washed and dried.

I couldn't help but notice the difficulties I faced in the kitchen. While I could wheel freely around the open space, reaching the cupboards and sink and the higher shelves in both the fridge and freezer proved to be challenging. Thankfully, my mother was there to assist me.

"It is nice to finally have you back home," my mother suggested, as we both sat at the kitchen table. "Although a little challenging, you must be happy to have this time outside of the rehab hospital."

"Lyndhurst is really not such a bad place. In fact, it grows on you. I tried to explain it to Dad on the way home this evening. It is so easy to become institutionalized by the comforts offered at Lyndhurst. There I am surrounded by others in wheelchairs, and the facilities are fully adapted to accommodate our needs. This trip home has shown me the reality of my circumstances, just how different I am now with a spinal cord injury. There will be no forgiveness when I face the real world. Preparing me for it is the best thing you and Dad can do right now."

It was a good feeling to be back as a family unit once again. I understood now what Colin meant by it being overwhelming at first, but he did say it would get better. I would have to take this move home one day at a time and not find my way back to the hospital so quickly. I would stick it out for at least the following day.

***

While my initial trip home brought a reality to my transitioning back into the real world I was quick to see the benefits of exposing myself to such an experience and continued my visits home on a more regular basis. It was early one Sunday morning, months later that I was at home in the kitchen with my mother when the telephone rang. We were well into November. With my home visits more frequent I was adjusting to using a wheelchair outside of Lyndhurst. I was also much stronger physically and no longer fully in need of my back brace. My father came into the kitchen to inform me the call was for me.

"Hi Wendy, it's Pat." It was Patricia O'Neill, Grania's mother.

I knew why she was calling. With mixed emotions I responded, "Yes Pat, I will definitely see you all today."

The O'Neill family had immigrated to Canada in the spring of 1976. It was said not to have been a difficult decision, the result of all the political turmoil in Northern Ireland around that time. They came as a family of seven: Patricia and Tony and the five children, Michael, Grania, Siobhan, Ciaran, and Joseph. They were a loving family with rules to be followed; not unlike most parents, Pat and Tony wanted the best for their five children. They were happy to be in a country free of political conflict, and they brought with them a work ethic many families would marvel at.

Pat O'Neill was pregnant at the time of the accident and as a result, she suffered from extreme anxiety, which could come on when she found herself in crowds or in some way confined. This often happened on the subway, which she had to ride downtown to and from work. When she was overwhelmed by what was happening, she often resorted to Grania to assist her. Grania would meet her on the subway line and help her get home. They were a very close mother-daughter team.

Three months after the accident, Pat gave birth to the O'Neill family's newest addition at Brampton Memorial Hospital. At close to seven and a half pounds, Fiona Patricia O'Neill came into the world a little after 9:00 am on November 2nd, 1984.

It was an emotional time on many levels. Grania's death had left a great void for us all, and I was still coming to terms with my own condition. Surviving the accident had originally appeared to be a blessing, but now, months later, full recuperation and regaining all my mobility no longer appeared promising. Grania's death was an ominous factor in this equation. However, Fiona's arrival brought with it a welcoming air of renewal. Many people considered it the offering of a new soul into what remained a very vacant reality, almost filling the hollowness that so often consumed many of us.

Fiona's baptism was to take place that Sunday morning and I was honoured to be asked to stand as her godmother.

I went to the church with my mom and dad. It had been some time since I had last attended mass, at least two weeks before the accident had occurred. My parents had left attending mass up to Kim and me after they gave us our Ford Mustang to share. I had occasionally attended Sunday evening mass with Grania.

Although we arrived at the church with plenty of time to spare (thanks to my father's habit of punctuality), a large crowd of neighbours and parishioners had gathered by the time we walked in the doors. The O'Neills were all there, seated at the front of the church. Shortly after arriving, I made my way over to where they were seated; Fiona looked darling.

I knew just how excited the family was to welcome this baby. All the O'Neill children were older, and this newcomer was a welcome surprise. But I also could not forget that Grania was no longer part of this reality; one she had longed to see happen. We had spoken endlessly about all that we would do with this newborn child. Despite the happiness about Fiona's birth, the reality of where things were today was less than joyful for me. I knew the family was sure to find the situation just as ambiguous.

As the baptism ceremony unfolded, I allowed myself to feel both emotions at once: sadness for the loss of my best friend, and joy for the arrival of the new life in the O'Neill family. Life does go on, and mine would too.

***

My days at Lyndhurst turned to weeks, which then turned to a number of months. I felt a comfort in this place, a kinship with the other patients who were here for rehabilitation. Unlike those in the general hospital, we were united in our purpose. Our goal was to gain physical strength and independence to enable us to return to mainstream society. Having all sustained spinal cord injuries through some form of trauma, many of us would now live life from a wheelchair permanently. Adapting to that reality was front and centre throughout our stay.

Our daily routine began with breakfast in the dining room, followed by mat class. Once my back brace was no longer needed and the doctors were confident the fusion of my spine was successful, I could take part in all the stretching and transfer training in mat class. These sessions were important for maintaining flexibility through stretching the body, which also increased blood flow through the paralyzed limbs.

The time available following mat class was usually open until lunch, giving me the opportunity to work independently in the gym with weights. This was often a time of reflection for me. Finding a routine in my schedule at Lyndhurst made it more likely that I would overcome all that had taken place and gain my independence and ability to face the real world once again. Getting around the hospital was never a problem, although I knew from my visits home that the real world outside of Lyndhurst would offer greater challenges. I hoped this would improve over time.

Lunch hour was traditionally a group activity. The actual people I shared a table with depended on where there was a place setting free, although Colin and I were always together. Our friendship had really evolved; both of us were paraplegic so we found ourselves with a lot in common in our physical limitations. While we both agreed we were more fortunate to have the use of our upper body, it was often difficult to accept the barriers we still faced.

Afternoons I spent one-on-one with my assigned physiotherapist, Martha, and our sessions were a welcome alternative to doing weights on my own. Range-of-motion exercise was a fulfilling activity now that sensation was returning to my legs. I could now feel the blood flow through my veins like a wild river, with few obstacles before meeting the open water. I looked forward to this and knew that things could only get better with time. My spinal cord was still healing, with more sensation likely to come. We also worked on strengthening my back and abdominal muscles, which were slowly reawakening. These muscles would assist me in sitting upright and reaching, while maintaining my balance.

I often rested in the later afternoon. Getting through the day without a nap took its toll, although my workouts were definitely paying off. I was much stronger now; so much so that Dr. Geisler mentioned my discharge during a visit to my room.

"Wendy, I've heard nothing but good things about the time you have put in at the gym," he began, "and the one-on-one physiotherapy sessions you have been having with Martha Binstock. This impresses me. Martha is not one to give praise very often."

"That is great to hear Dr. Geisler. I did give you my word that I would focus my efforts. I'm a girl of my word. What I say I'll do, I'm sure to do."

"Martha has also told us that she believes it's only a matter of weeks before you're ready to be discharged from her physio sessions."

"We certainly worked well as a team," I responded. "Her knowledge and guidance helped me in every area, particularly with my endurance."

"That's great to hear. Martha has been here at the hospital for quite some time now. She's gained incredible insights into spinal cord recovery and what can be achieved through proper treatment."

"She was also instrumental in keeping my expectations realistic," I pointed out.

"How is that, Wendy?"

"Well Dr. Geisler, since my diagnosis was an incomplete injury, I often hoped of one day walking again. That hope became stronger when sensation began to return."

"I can understand that, Wendy, although it was made clear to you that a spinal cord injury is very difficult to diagnose. There were no promises made. I am sure you've had the opportunity to meet some of your fellow in-patients, and you know that you have regained your former physical state more than many have."

While this was hard to hear, he was right. I had full use of my upper body, offering me much more physical independence than many, with the return of my feeling an added advantage. I had family, who were present and fully supportive throughout my recovery, with a new home in the works. Finally, there was my discharge from Lyndhurst Hospital, which now appeared to be a close reality. While all would have to meet as a team – doctor, physiotherapist, psychologist, and assigned nurse, I could now see my way through the forest. Going home was the primary objective now.

"I suppose you're right, Doctor, and I do my best to remain in that reality. It doesn't take away the loss I do feel. I was once very physically active, and this has been a real adjustment."

After I had expressed my thoughts so openly, Dr. Geisler didn't seem to know what to say. He had rounds to do throughout the hospital and graciously excused himself from the conversation.

Dr. Geisler's visit was brief, but it helped me come to terms with all that now was, and what would soon be. While a little voice deep down inside had been hoping I would see a full recovery at Lyndhurst and would walk again, I now knew that would not be the case. I still had a lot to be grateful for, and that included a discharge date that seemed possible in the not-too-distant future.

Chapter 7: Planning Lyndhurst Discharge

After months of rehabilitation at Lyndhurst Hospital, I was finding my way around life confined to a wheelchair. I had come to terms with living while facing obstacles from all directions. However, I was unsure of just how bearable those changes and challenges would become after I left the security of Lyndhurst.

I was feeling grateful for all my family was willing to do to accommodate the circumstances. A family counsellor and a psychologist were put on my patient care case, and it was during a family session that we were told our home would not be suitable for my wheelchair. Our house was a split-level style, with stairs necessary to get to all levels. The family counsellor suggested I could find a place to live on my own after I was discharged, rather than forcing my family to move into a new home. The thought of this scared me. I was hardly prepared to take on a fully independent lifestyle; there was so much to adapt to, and many obstacles to face while trying to adjust to living in a wheelchair. I had not lived outside our family home before the accident, and I certainly felt I was in no position to take on such a move now. I did not see it my place to make the decision for my parents, hardly wanting them to move with regrets, blaming the transition on me.

In the end, my parents insisted that a move to a more accommodating house would be the best choice, for my adjustment to living at home and for all of us.

The home we were able to purchase was adapted so that my wheelchair would have full access. There were standards and codes that had to be followed to ensure I could get to all parts of the home, with a safe exit in case of an emergency such as fire. An elevator would be installed through the garage to bring me to the entry level, as well as to the master bedroom and basement.

When the home was purchased, we consulted with engineers and our real estate agent, Sean Yeates, and decided that since my access through the garage would take me straight into the master bedroom, it stood to reason that I would take possession of it. The room also had a private bathroom that better suited my needs, with a wider door and pedestal sink. No renovations would have to be done to that bathroom. The master bedroom and bathroom were move-in ready, although the elevator installation was a must before I could return home.

One morning, I had just finished physiotherapy when I was paged to the front reception desk of the hospital. I was tired and wondered who wanted me at the entrance. Entering the lobby, I saw my father standing at reception, grinning from ear to ear.

"Wendy, I have great news. The renovations are coming along and we think you'll be in good hands with us all as a family come your discharge date. We're looking at a couple of weeks from now."

"A couple of weeks! That's not much time to prepare, Dad. Are you sure it's a realistic time frame?"

My father appeared confused. I had constantly pushed for a discharge date through my medical team, and now that the date appeared close, I was having second thoughts.

"Well Wendy, it's been your impatience in the past that has us all hoping to make this work sooner rather than later. Are you telling me you're okay remaining here in the hospital?"

I did not know how to respond to that. My thoughts were mixed.

"I'm not saying it can't happen but I do question a two-week time frame. There's my supplies and medications to be ordered. Is everybody prepared to have me at home with the renovations not yet finished?"

I was scrambling for excuses. Although I was looking forward to being discharged, I wasn't sure that I was ready to face the real world just yet. I would miss many things when I actually left, including the friends I had made, as well as the security, comforts, and access at Lyndhurst. I knew that there would be more obstacles to face once I was outside the hospital.

My trips home on weekends had given me a feel for the attitudes and difficulties I would face, and my mind was now racing with the reality of it all. While some areas of society were changing where accessibility was concerned, communities for the most part still needed work. Whether it was entering and exiting a building, gaining access to a second floor, or most importantly, the washrooms, people in wheelchairs were often at a huge disadvantage. This made any significant time spent in these less accessible places very tense.

"Wendy, your mother and I have tried to make it clear to you that we are all here to assist you through your transition but don't underestimate the changes we've taken on since the accident. It's been difficult on us all. We've been with you from the beginning and it can take a toll."

"I'm sorry, Dad, the last thing I want is to sound ungrateful for all that you have done. But it comes down to whether I feel ready to make a full-time commitment."

"It would seem you've forgotten the golden rule of your recovery," my father said. "Taking things one day at a time. I suggest that if you find a way to keep your mind on that rule, we'll all get through this. Prolonging the inevitable will not change the reality. You'll have to be discharged at some point."

His words were reassuring; words only a caring father could share, although I could not get past my apprehension at actually leaving Lyndhurst. There was so much for me to face while trying to move forward with my life, I was not sure I would succeed. It was like starting life all over again, with a wheelchair now in the picture. What would my life be like? How difficult an adjustment would this actually be? I knew my father was right. I might never feel comfortable facing the unknown. I would have to give it my best effort, just as all the members of my family had.

My physiotherapy had reached a plateau at Lyndhurst. I still attended mat class regularly in the mornings, with weights and pulleys my focus in the afternoon. I was still under the care of physiotherapist Martha Binstock, who had brought me further than anyone would have anticipated. My upper body strength had improved enormously; I could now transfer myself in and out of my wheelchair independently, even when using a bathtub and toilet. The one transfer that remained a challenge was getting from the wheelchair into a car, with family and friends usually needed to assist. I also struggled with my floor-to-wheelchair lifts (getting from the floor into my wheelchair). I found the lift to be much too strenuous, and decided it was one manoeuvre I would need help with for now.

I made my way back to my room while my father hunted down the social worker to inquire about the arrangements that would have to be made before I could go home permanently. There were supplies to be ordered, medications to be prescribed and filled, and home renovations to finish before I could feel fully confident leaving the hospital.

Not long after I got back to my room, I was joined by Angie.

"There you are," she said. "I've been looking all over for you. I've got great news to share! It would appear I'm finally breaking free of this place. That's right, I have my discharge date and I'm thrilled to know I'll finally be on a plane and heading back home. Can you believe it?"

"That's great news, Angie. How much longer will you be sharing your lovely smile with the rest of us here at Lyndhurst?" I asked.

I knew I was also on my way out, perhaps before her, but I decided I would not mention my own planned departure. I thought it would be best to wait and see what the medical team would decide for my discharge date. This had me a little concerned, given the amount of help I had been able to offer Angie when the nurses were simply too busy. How would she cope without me if I left first?

"It looks like I'll be leaving the middle of next month. I hope you'll find a way to get along without me here."

"Well Angie, there's little doubt you will be missed. How do you feel about returning to Thunder Bay and rejoining your family?" I asked.

"I feel torn. That's the best way to describe it. It's been a long haul for me since my transfer from Thunder Bay. While I know coming here was the best thing for my recovery, losing the support of my family and friends took some getting used to. I was grateful to be welcomed by a new group here at the hospital, but it's been lonely at times not to have my family closer. I'm looking forward to reuniting with them."

Oddly enough, I could relate to what Angie was saying. Although her stay at Lyndhurst was certainly longer than mine, we had all found a way to bond through our shared experiences. While some of us were less challenged, depending on the level of our injuries, we could all relate to each other through the spinal damage we had suffered.

My father entered the room and walked over to where we were sitting, close to Angie's side of the room. The drapes were pulled back, offering an open view of the grounds that surrounded the hospital.

"Well hello ladies, I hope I'm not interrupting anything too important," he asked. "I assume you are both getting ready for dinner. Wendy, what do you say we eat together in the visitor's cafeteria downstairs? I have a few things to discuss with you."

I immediately knew that my father had spoken to someone on my medical team. The question was, what had been discussed and with whom?

We headed down to the basement of the hospital where the public cafeteria was located. It was Friday, which meant fish and chips, a big favourite of mine. We made our way with our trays over to an empty table located close to the cafeteria lounge. I began with my questions almost immediately.

"So how did it go with my medical team this afternoon? Was anything decided?"

"I was able to get an appointment with Lauren Brady, your social worker, and we discussed a discharge date," said my father.

"You may never feel that you are fully prepared to leave this facility and all the security it offers, but we can't postpone the inevitable. We are now living in our new home. There's no real reason why you shouldn't join us."

"I just worry about my daily workouts. The facilities here have brought me so far."

"They've decided that you've reached your highest level of recovery, and coming home is the next step for you. It's time to make your bed here at rehab available for others who need it."

My father was right. While I was worried about whether I was ready for discharge from Lyndhurst, prolonging the actual move would do no one any good.

Angie faced much more of an adjustment with her discharge than I did. She had hundreds of miles to travel, to a home that was yet to be fully adapted to her needs. We had discussed what she felt her return home would be like and there was little doubt she was prepared to face a different mentality than you would find in a bigger city like Toronto. She had received cards and letters that often reflected what many back home believed to be her future. Some could not see all that she could still accomplish while sitting in a power wheelchair. Some were encouraging, but many conveyed a sense of empathy that Angie felt uncomfortable accepting.

With her spinal cord damaged at level C5, 6, she was paralyzed from her shoulders down, limiting her arm and hand movements. But she was a very strong-willed individual. Her sights were set on returning to university, and I was confident she could do it. She was a spitfire, a real trouper when it came to applying herself. That included everything she did to better herself through her physiotherapy sessions. If she was told to do ten minutes of pulleys, Angie would do fifteen. If it was suggested she be at Occupational Therapy for two o'clock in the afternoon, she'd arrive at 1:45 and work on any activity that would improve her resilience to the challenges she was now forced to face without the full use of her hands. Whether it was creating colourful characters with play dough or stuffing envelopes, Angie was practising what she could still do with her hands, in hope of improvement.

Suddenly my situation felt less dire. And after speaking with Angie, there was a side of me much more ready to depart the four walls that for so long had been my strength and encouragement. Unlike her, I had enjoyed the comforts of my family throughout my stay, with visits home on weekends. If anyone was ready for discharge, it should be me. And while I did face limitations, there would be no comparing who was better off, mobility wise.

"I suppose you are right, Dad. Going home is the right move to make in my recovery," I finally agreed.

Chapter 8: Newfound Freedom

With my physiotherapy reaching a plateau and my discharge from Lyndhurst a foreseeable reality, preparation for life outside of rehab was now on the agenda. I'd have to purchase things like a personal, custom fit wheelchair, a sliding board for transfers, and finally everyday supplies such as catheters and medications. The one aspect of my independence I had not gained at Lyndhurst Hospital would be getting back in the driver's seat – driving a vehicle.

The Hugh MacMillan Centre was offering driving lessons to those wanting to reintroduce themselves to the practice of driving a car. This process would now be mastered through the use of hand controls, a brilliant alternative for those unable to use their legs. There are bars attached to both the gas and brake pedals, requiring the driver to pull down on the lever for gas, and to push in on the lever for brakes.

It all began when Lindsay, my occupational therapist, scheduled an appointment with driving instructor David Kennedy.

There were many questions running through my head. I could not fathom just how I'd be able to drive without the use of my legs. I was about to find out.

"Hi Wendy, so glad you could make the appointment," were David's first words.

"Yes, and so am I ... I think."

"You sound hesitant about that, Wendy."

"Well, I do have a few questions about driving a vehicle now that I am paralyzed from the waist down. I don't quite see how that would be possible, David."

"If you'll follow me, I'll put your curiosity to rest."

I accompanied David down a long corridor and into a room at the end of the hall. The room was larger than I had expected, with a piece of equipment sitting front and centre. David went over to it and invited me to join him. At that point he explained the miraculous and very functional piece of equipment I was looking at.

"Wendy, this is a simulator. It has been designed as a piece of training equipment for those paralyzed but still hoping to drive a motor vehicle. These are the hand controls. Come on over and get behind the wheel."

Moving closer to David I could see the steering wheel and the hand control, which was a straight bar located just under the steering wheel, on the left side. One thing was clear, you could not use hand controls on a car with standard transmission; your left hand was busy with the gas and brake and your right hand was used to steer. Driving a standard would be impossible.

David grabbed a chair and sat in front of the simulator.

"As I explained, this is a simulator. Its purpose is to give you a feel for what the hand controls will be like in an actual car. It's a fairly simple transition. We'll be taking the car out later this morning, after I see you are comfortable working with the hand controls we have set up here."

"You mean I will be going out in a car today?!"

I was hesitant. Although it had been some time since the accident, there was a big part of me still very anxious when it came to driving, or even being a passenger in a car. I could not forget what had happened to me and my worries something might happen again grew stronger the more I had anything to do with cars, especially when driving on the highways.

"Of course we'll work on your skills with the simulator. Once I feel you're ready, taking the car out along the side streets is common practice. Are you ready for this, Wendy?"

Not wanting to discourage him, and knowing I would have to get past this before my discharge from Lyndhurst, I agreed to his terms.

"Yes, yes, of course I am ready for this. It will be a piece of cake …
a walk in the park. Make some space for me to get in there. Let's get
this show on the road," I said, trying to sound more confident than I
felt.

"Now that's what I like to hear. I'm confident you will see that
the technique is fairly straightforward."

He moved aside to allow me to pull my wheelchair in front of
the simulator.

"There you have the hand control on your left. Pull it down,
using moderate force. That is how you activate the gas pedal. Pretty
easy, wouldn't you say, Wendy?"

"That's it? I pull the lever down to accelerate. I'd say that is a
fairly simple process. Now how do I stop?" I asked.

"Just as simply. You are going to push in the hand control to
apply the brakes. Go ahead Wendy, give it a try."

Following David's instruction I gently pushed in on the lever
and watched the brake on the simulator compress. This was
fantastic, I thought. And what freedom it could offer.

"You weren't kidding when you said I'd pick up on this, it's a
very straightforward process."

"We'll have you test through a few simulated neighbourhoods
before we actually take you out on the road. I have a good sense that
you'll pick up on these hand controls no problem, and that we'll be
taking you out on the road at some point this afternoon."

I was initially uncomfortable by the thought of taking a car back
on the road. While I had been a passenger in motor vehicles since
the accident, taking control of one felt like a daunting task, one I was
not thoroughly sure I wanted to take on. I attempted to postpone
the inevitable.

"Does it all have to happen today?" I asked.

"No Wendy, not at all, although my appointments are backed
up until this coming fall. It was my understanding that you wanted
to put this process behind you before your discharge from
Lyndhurst."

His words were so affirming that I had to agree. I did wish to
have this over with before I went home for good. There would be

less reason to have to return to the hospital. It would also put me that much further toward a fully independent lifestyle. Now was not the time to put any of this on hold.

"You're right," I responded. "This was my hope, so let's get through it."

David came over to where I was sitting in front of the simulator and walked me through all the things I would need to know. The precautions included giving the hand control the right amount of pressure to accelerate the gas to move the car forward while in drive, not putting too much pressure on the brakes when initiating a stop, how to turn on the signal while steering the car, and finally, adjusting all the mirrors properly to try and ensure I had full view outside of the vehicle.

"It looks like you have the technique down, Wendy," said David after we had been through all the steps. "What do you say we take you outside and onto some of the side streets around here? It will give you a good run at actually driving while not exposing either one of us to any danger. It's a natural progression to begin on the closer roads."

I was anxious to resume my place behind the wheel, and I knew that facing my fear was the first step.

"Sure, David. I'm dead set on driving again, so I suppose getting out there on the road is the only way I'll see past this."

"That's a good way of looking at it. I'll take you through the preliminary stages, which we've begun this morning. The road test after the simulator is where things go from here. I'll evaluate your abilities on the road, how you manage the vehicle. Ultimately, you will have to redo your road test at the Ministry of Transportation."

Oh great, I thought. I had been a bag of nerves the *first time* I'd taken my test, and that was while I was able-bodied. Being tested now with hand controls would only add to the torture.

After some practice both David and I proceeded out to the parking lot to a waiting yellow Ford, an older model car with radial tires, complete with four doors and a cloth interior. I couldn't help but react to the car.

"I don't know that I'll get far before being stopped, given the state of what I'll be driving. Are you sure this thing has passed its road inspections?"

"It's not style and luxury we're aiming for here, it's safe and practical features, and this car will offer both. It's trained a number of individuals on the transition to hand controls. It serves its purpose."

I transferred myself into the driver's side of the car while David collapsed the wheelchair, placing it into the trunk. He then joined me on the bench seat of the car while I slowly buckled up the seat belt, preparing myself for my first drive behind the wheel since before the accident. I felt a confused state of excitement mixed with a restless anxiety. How will I do this again? I thought. How safe will I be behind the wheel or on the roads? While I was confident in my knowledge of the rules of the road, how easy it would be to apply them while driving with hand controls was another concern.

"You're one of my many students taking on this initial attempt, Wendy, and I am confident that you too will catch on to this concept with little difficulty. It's getting started that takes courage. Once we're out there on the road you'll pick up on it, I'm sure."

"I'm glad you have faith in me. We'll soon see just how right you are," I responded.

We decided I would get familiar with the hand controls by driving around the parking lot. My first test came with starting the car. I knew to pull down on the lever to accelerate the gas, so all went well there. Next step was to brake the car while I shifted into drive. It felt like no time before we were moving freely around the somewhat deserted parking area. After only a few turns around the grounds I felt I was ready to try the road.

"Well David, I guess you were right when you said I would catch on to this. I believe I'm ready to try the roadway now, so long as we remain on the side streets."

"Yes, from what I'm seeing you are definitely prepared to test your skills outside of these facilities. If you drive around those parked cars we'll come to the exit. The streets around this place will be just what you need for practice before we hit any of the more congested roadways."

I entered the street cautiously, with both hands tightly gripping the hand control lever and the steering wheel. The speed limit was forty kilometres per hour, and I was sure to stay at or below that speed. We travelled through the neighbourhood for fifteen or twenty minutes before David decided we were ready to take things to the next level. That would mean taking us out on the much busier roads, with higher speed limits as well as lane changes and stop lights.

"You can take a right-hand turn at the next stop sign, Wendy. I believe Bayview Avenue would be a good place to begin a short trip through the city. There'll be enough traffic lights and left-turn lanes to test your abilities with the hand controls. The higher speed limit will also be good for you."

Following David's direction I made my way onto Bayview Avenue and almost immediately felt the stresses of the road. Cars were whizzing past me, horns began to beep, and my blood pressure began to rise.

"My God, David, are you certain I'm ready for this? I feel like I'm on an Indy racetrack. I'm willing to turn back if you are."

"No, no, Wendy, you're doing fine. Just stay here in the outside lane, and we'll get you accustomed to the speed of the road. We won't begin testing your turning skills until you feel comfortable. Trust me, your confidence will return," David assured me.

My thoughts suddenly deepened as I realized all that was happening, and my comfort zone began to shrink. My God, I thought, I am back on the road and behind the wheel. Suddenly my adrenaline rose as my confidence dwindled. The cars continued to pass us while I did my best to keep us safely on the road.

"You're doing just fine, Wendy. We are on these roads at a good time, with less congestion. Now, at the second set of lights I'd like you to put your left indicator on while we attempt your first left turn."

David's reassurance really helped the situation. I could feel myself getting calmer, and my concentration became sharper.

It felt like mere seconds before we were face to face with the left-turn lane, and with my indicator on I ventured into the lane cautiously, stopping behind the car ahead of me as we waited for the light to turn green. It was to my advantage that there was an advanced green light, offering me the opportunity to make it through safely. Something told me that David was fully aware of this blessing as I gradually accelerated by pulling down on the hand control lever, following the blue Dodge ahead of me. It seemed no time before we were through the middle of the intersection and safely back on the neighbourhood side street. I was able to bring the car to a full stop, eager to hear more on the progress I had made.

"David you really had me worked up out there. Do you push all of your students this hard? How did I do?" I asked.

"I knew you'd do well. I have a good eye for those who can coordinate the gas pedal from the brake while adjusting to the hand control. I was confident while watching you work on the simulator, and my intuition was confirmed when I took you out on the road.

"Wendy, many of my students are recent injuries who've driven for a while before they need to use the hand controls. I consider myself a refresher course for those who are familiar with the rules of the road. The controls are not that hard to pick up on. If I left it up to some of my students, though, we might never graduate to the actual roads. Many are initially apprehensive."

"Thanks for your vote of trust when you took me out onto Bayview Avenue. I was taken aback at first, but I guess things calmed the more I drove."

"I'm glad you were able to overcome your nervousness because our class is not over yet. Before you can be considered certified, you'll have to master parking this beast. Let's move the car forward and attempt to parallel park between those two cars up ahead."

"Parallel park! I could hardly do that using my feet on the pedals and two hands on the steering wheel," I exclaimed.

I was anything but pleased to hear my parking skills would now be tested. When I was an able-bodied driver I used to park blocks away to avoid having to attempt such a daunting task. How was I expected to accomplish this using hand controls?

"Come on now, I have tremendous faith in your abilities after that drive we shared down Bayview Avenue. Don't question yourself now, Wendy. Just pull up beside that red four-door vehicle and we'll test your parking skills from there," was David's response.

Not in any mood to argue, I followed his direction, driving the car directly beside the red Ford before preparing to back the tail end of the car into the available space. As both my hands were occupied, I felt confined, with no way to move to get a clear view of where the rear of the car was heading. I was unable to see much by simply turning my head in either direction. This had me totally dependent on the rear and side view mirrors.

"Well," I blurted, "this won't be easy at all...."

"The mirrors will be your guide, Wendy. Are they positioned properly for you? Do you have a clear vision as to where you want to aim the back end of the car?"

"Yes," I responded. But I realized that parking the car using two feet had been a much easier task.

I began backing the rear of the car into the space available. On my first try I failed hopelessly. I was relieved that David had found a very quiet street for me to practise on. I moved the car forward to try again, and again, no luck. At that point, David agreed to get out of the car and better direct me into the space. Using all accessible mirrors, and through the meticulous direction of my instructor, my efforts proved more successful. I made it into the parking space with great precision.

With the major road test completed and the parallel parking task achieved, our session was considered a success. I drove us safely back to the Hugh MacMillan Centre before rush hour traffic began, which made it a much less stressful drive for us both. Upon our arrival back at the Centre, David offered words of encouragement.

"Well Wendy, I can assure you you've caught on to this concept of mobility impressively," he said as he retrieved my wheelchair from the trunk of the car. "I've been assessing individuals with the simulator and road tests for quite some time now, and I have to say you were quick at picking up the hand controls. I don't see you having much problem with the transition, other than practising a little more with the parallel parking. It's not guaranteed that you'll be tested on that task when you go for your driver's license, although a little more practice couldn't hurt. The skill will certainly come in handy."

"You're right about the parking," I replied. "Although it's a task I could avoid, it might make life a little easier if I worked on it."

It had been five months now since the accident, and this driving test brought everything back to the surface. I had come full circle in my rehab. Because of my paralysis, driving a car once again was not a skill I had ever contemplated. In fact, most of what I learned while at Lyndhurst showed me how I could resume my life in so many ways. While there would definitely be challenges, I would continue to face them head on. I could see now that there was so much to be grateful for, a lot to live for, and the onus was on me to see the glass half full. Thanks to the time I had spent at Lyndhurst Hospital I now had the personal means to move forward with my life.

Chapter 9: Coming Home

It was with mixed feelings that I accepted my time at Lyndhurst was up. The next stage of my recovery would be moving back with the family. I was excited to know that I would no longer be a patient, but now a normal member of society hoping to mainstream back into society. But after having been hospitalized for more than seven months, I was also faced with doubt. How could I hope to fit in to a world no longer fully welcoming to my physical abilities? What could I hope to achieve while trying to adapt?

When the day finally arrived to leave Lyndhurst and go home for good, I knew that one way or another all my questions would find answers.

My family had purchased a new home in our existing neighbourhood. Both my parents were active members in Our Lady of the Airways Parish, and it made sense to stay near the community that was such a vital part of our transition. Our new home was a two-storey house with a living room, dining room, four bedrooms, four bathrooms, a spacious family room, and a finished basement. The real treat for me was gaining my own bedroom. My sister and I had always shared a room, but that would now change. I would take the elevator directly up into the master bedroom.

"Hello Wendy, and welcome," called my mother as I transferred myself from car to wheelchair, my father proudly observing the independence that I was clearly displaying. "It's such a pleasure to finally have you home with us, dear."

"Thanks, Mom, the pleasure is truly mine," I responded without hesitating. I could hardly believe that I was actually home for good, the months of hospitals behind me now.

Both my sister, Kim, and brother, Jeff, had just gotten home when I arrived, and this made for an intimate introduction to my new surroundings. We entered the home using the elevator, which had been installed so that its entrance was accessible from the two-car garage.

The elevator gave me full access to our home. My tour began on the main level.

"Wow, I never would have imagined things to be so well thought out and implemented. From the looks of things I have full access to this house, and I feel much more at ease seeing it first-hand."

"Wendy, it's through the efforts of some knowledgeable people that we were able to find this home. We purchased it only after we were assured the modifications could be done."

"They've done very well!" was my response.

"Concord Elevator is responsible for the lift, and the emergency exit ramp around the backyard is new, but the rest of the house we purchased as is. It simply suited our needs," my father added as I explored the main level of the house.

I was very pleased with what I saw. Suddenly my sister's voice echoed through the hallway.

"Wendy, there's much more to see up here!"

"Mom, Dad, please take me upstairs!" I asked.

"Dear, this is your home now," my mother responded. "I'm sure you'll have no problem getting yourself upstairs in the elevator. Go on, join your sister."

As I made my way into the elevator, I was thrilled to be home. Not just in any home, but in our home, a home that would now facilitate my mobility. The engineers who had designed the modifications were brilliant. It seemed there would be no boundaries for me here. I was elated to witness all that my family had accomplished the months I spent preparing for my discharge, not realizing they too were hard at work. They often referred to the renovations that were going on behind the scenes but I would never have anticipated such a seamless transition.

I joined my sister in the master bedroom, my new bedroom. She appeared just as excited as I was for me to finally be home.

"Wendy, can you believe it? Your days with hospitals are over. It's so great to have you home!"

"And so great to be here!"

The excitement we shared was palpable. I made my way around the room taking it all in slowly. The closet wall had been knocked out and replaced with sliding mirror doors. This gave me full access to my clothing and the storage bins stacked to the left. There was a full bathroom right off the bedroom that also offered me barrier-free access, unlike the master bathroom off the hallway that would be used by the rest of the family. I moved in and out of each room on the upstairs level offering my stamp of approval before exiting.

"Now onto the basement!" my sister commanded. "Bet I'll beat you there!"

I quickly headed back into the elevator, bound for the basement. It was a slow trip, eliminating any chance of me arriving there before Kim. While going down my thoughts turned to just how lucky I was to have the love and support of my family, all that they had done to make my discharge possible. I am truly blessed, I thought.

"Over here!" I heard as I exited the lift and made my way into the basement. My sister was pointing out the accessible bathroom, complete with a Jacuzzi bathtub.

The tour of the home was incredible and put to rest any doubts I had about my discharge. While I had become used to doing things in a routine fashion during the months I spent in rehabilitation, I was home now and ready to establish new routines. There would be no more morning gatherings in the dining room at Lyndhurst with the others, which was a start to the day I had always looked forward to.

Topics of conversation always varied and it was the time shared together that really made the difference. We were all working toward a common goal, to regain our independence and find our way back into some form of productive role outside of Lyndhurst Hospital. I would actually miss mat class now. Although I had found many of the transfers I practised during the class to be challenging at times, the class offered me a place to improve on what would be necessary to live independently when I was outside of the comfort zone that Lyndhurst created. Although I didn't realize it at the time, having everything perfectly designed at Lyndhurst to facilitate our wheelchairs could be a detriment due to the challenges we would face when we attempted to move on outside of the facility. And finally, my daily physiotherapy sessions with Martha were now over. Although I could continue to do workouts independently now that I was at home, I would not have her enthusiasm and encouragement to push me on when I felt at my wits' end during workouts. How could I be sure my discipline wouldn't fail? How could I continue to the best of my ability?

Not wanting to take away from the excitement, I suggested we join the rest of the family on the main level. My father was busy taking in the bags from the car while my mother called me into the kitchen, a kitchen I now had full access to.

"There'll be no more struggles for you here, Wendy," she said. "We are so happy that we were able to adapt things for you here."

"I couldn't be happier, Mom, although I'm anxious to think I'm one step closer to living independently. While I did most of my personal care while at the rehab centre, knowing the staff was there did offer reassurance, and I'm feeling a little vulnerable right now."

"That is understandable, dear. You've been under the care of doctors and nurses who all agree this is the best move for you. You have us all here as a family to support you now."

"I know you're right. I guess I'm just a little edgy about it all. I am thrilled to be home though, and to such a beautiful home."

I hoped that the honesty I shared about my anxious feelings would not put a damper on all that was happening. I was finally in our new family home, purchased specifically to facilitate my needs. I knew there was no turning back. There was a lot to look forward to now that I had been discharged, with family life now more in focus. Something that had seemed impossible months earlier was now actually happening. And strangely, I felt it was something I was ready to face, despite the restless feelings.

Not long after making my way into the kitchen with my mother, we were joined by the rest of the family.

"Well, what do you think, Wendy, have we lived up to your expectations?" My father asked.

"Funny you should ask, Dad. I'm moved by all the efforts put into completing the renovations. I couldn't ask for a more barrier-free environment. I hope you haven't sacrificed too much to accommodate my needs."

My sister was the first to jump in.

"Are you kidding? This house is a far cry from living in our old split level. We each have our own bedroom now!"

I agreed with Kim, although it was my parents I was hoping to hear from. I wondered whether they had faced any financial burdens with the real estate purchase.

It was then that my mother suggested I go to the refrigerator and get out some fresh lettuce. She was going to begin preparing dinner for that evening. I was reassured to see there would be few barriers for me anywhere around the kitchen.

"I have to thank you all as a family," I began. "There's no way to truly describe just how welcome I feel to be home, in our new home."

"We are family, Wendy. We would not want it any other way," my mother assured me.

Both my mother and I got busy in the kitchen preparing dinner, and it was when all the family finally sat down to eat that I was able to share my reflective thoughts with them.

"I really meant what I said earlier. I am tremendously grateful for all that you've done as a family to help my transition. I have only been home a short time but I feel this is going to work. I'm determined to see myself through this and I am very thankful for the sacrifices you've made to see me this far. I hope you all know that."

"Yes, of course we do. Your mother and I said from the beginning, Wendy, that although it would test us as a family, we would see you through this."

"I suppose it was seeing the difficulties many of the other patients faced," I said. "Whether it was the physical challenges they were adjusting to or seeing their family unit fall to pieces. You have shined through this, not only in your support through my rehab, but actually moving into this new home for me. I feel truly blessed."

My bother Jeff jumped in to the conversation.

"What did you expect us to do? We love you, big sister!"

"Well, you've certainly shown that, little brother, in more ways than you know," I responded. "There was so much I saw that made me appreciate my own situation. I could see that almost immediately after arriving at the Centre."

"Seeing the glass half full is the better way to get through most challenges, dear," said my mother. "The fact that we could help you as a family is testament to our love for you. We would not dare turn our backs at a time so crucial."

The most rewarding part of the evening was sitting down to a home cooked meal. My mother's culinary abilities were never more obvious to me after having relied on hospital food for all those months. While the food at Lyndhurst was prepared by a chef, no one could come close to my mother's cooking.

After dinner, I did another tour of the house with my sister and brother. I could not get over all that they had thought of and how perfect it all seemed.

My first evening home was a real awakening for me in many aspects of my life. I was now home and not in a holding pattern at Lyndhurst waiting for accessible housing to move to. My family had purchased a new home for me, adapting it according to my needs. Then there was my condition and all that I remained able to do for myself like dressing and taking on my own personal care including washing, brushing my teeth, and doing my hair and makeup when need be. Things appeared to be looking up. But would I succeed independently, was the question. I could not get past the thought of not having the nurses around to assist me if I needed help. And would my independence be impeded now? Would I need the help of others, now that I was home?

I headed up to bed later that night concerned that I would not succeed at adapting to my new surroundings. I took the elevator up from the main level and into my bedroom. The atmosphere was serene while I got ready for bed, something I hardly ever felt while at Lyndhurst, sharing my room with three other patients. Bedtime could be a very confusing time with each one of us in need of some form of help. The confusion was high at times. Not tonight: I had the whole room to myself, complete with a private bathroom. My duties began with a change of clothes, from street clothes to pajamas. I struggled a little with the pajama bottoms but did not call in my mom or sister to assist me. I accomplished the task on my own. After washing, the real chore was getting into bed independently. While my transfers were not a problem when moving onto a level surface, my bed was quite a hike higher than my wheelchair. I made sure that both brakes were on before lifting myself up and over, with extra lift necessary to ensure I made it onto the bed. Surprisingly, I made it up. With that achieved there was nothing left to conquer, other than to sleep.

I woke the following morning startled in my new environment. The curtains usually draped around my bed at Lyndhurst to offer privacy were nowhere in sight, and the room I now found myself in was very spacious. Not long after waking I was joined by my mother, who knocked before entering the room.

"Good morning, Wendy. While I was beside myself to see you this morning I didn't want to wake you. I do hope you realize just how nice it is to have you home with us?"

"Thanks, Mom. I still feel like I need a pinch to ensure it's actually happening, it seems so surreal. I've imagined this homecoming so many times in my mind that I could almost taste it. Seeing it all unfold has been so pleasurable."

"Your father and I told you many times it would all work out in the end, didn't we? You've come so far in your recovery, but it's family time that you need now."

"I know, you're right there, Mom. Only a few months ago I couldn't see myself outside of a bed. I've come a long way thanks to the rehab at Lyndhurst."

"You've come a long way thanks to the incredible strength you have shown, dear. I don't think you realize that."

"I suppose, but to see all those patients at Lyndhurst with less mobility than I have … now that's strength. I feel blessed in many ways."

It was a touching moment of reflection and I was pleased to have had that time with my mother. There seemed to be so much going on with my return home those intimate times were often missed. I was so privileged to be surrounded by the love and support of my family that I felt I could overcome anything. My future was now up to me.

My first full day home was dedicated to transitioning to home life. I had all my belongings to organize and move into my new bedroom. The family had completed the initial move; I now had to find a place for all of it. It's sometimes mind boggling how when you put a room full of stuff into boxes: it appears to double the actual amount on hand. Looking around the room at the boxes full to the top, I hardly knew where to start. There were clothes, books, shoes, dancing awards ... the list was endless. I spent most of the day in my room attempting to make it more presentable. Later in the afternoon my sister joined me to fill me in on plans for later that evening.

"Hey Wendy, you have really done a lot in here," my sister commented as she entered the bedroom.

"Thanks for noticing, it's certainly been a lot of work. I've been in here all day."

"Sounds like you could use a night out, and I know just the thing."

"What are you hinting at, Kim? It certainly sounds intriguing."

"There's a group going out to Fifty Second Street tonight and I thought you might like to join them."

Fifty Second Street was a local bar that my sister and many of her friends would frequent on weekends to eat, drink, and enjoy some dancing. I had visited it prior to the accident, using my sister Kim's identification. She was older than me and at the legal age to drink. I had celebrated my nineteenth birthday while in the Toronto Western Hospital. Dr. Wright actually prescribed me a Molson Export beer that evening, as my first legal alcoholic beverage. I was now of legal age to venture out to the bars and night clubs, although doing so in a wheelchair would come with challenges, given the crowds often found in these establishments.

"Sure! I'd love to join everyone. What time were they planning on meeting there?" I asked.

"Any time after seven o'clock, I'll let them know we'll be joining them!"

I was pleased with what I was able to accomplish that day. My room now reflected me and my new journey in life. With the closet adapted to facilitate my wheelchair my clothes were more accessible, and my bathroom was also ready to accommodate my needs.

Knowing we would be eating out I skipped dinner and opted for some cheese with crackers, something to subdue my appetite until we all made it to Fifty Second Street. Knowing the venue, I pulled out jeans and a jean shirt to wear with a pair of flat bone-coloured booties and a matching belt. My wardrobe would now have to adjust to my condition. I now purchased jeans one size up, a 27-inch waistline instead of 26 inches to allow for comfort; boots would now have to be flat due to a fusion of my left tibia; all in all a few minor adjustments given the circumstances. My hair was just below shoulder length and I pulled it back into a ponytail for the evening. I joined my sister in the family room before our departure.

"Well I'm ready anytime you are, Kim."

"And looking great I might add. I'm so glad you've agreed to join us tonight."

"I've been out of the loop for a long time. It's just what I need to get me more in tune with the real world now that I am home for good."

My sister and I made our way to the bar and were greeted by a large lineup when we arrived. To my surprise, we were ushered up to the front of the line immediately. Wow, I thought, this wheelchair can have beneficial perks too.

We met up with our group as soon as we got inside. Jane and Christine Smith were the first to approach us.

"Kim, Wendy, we're all sitting over there by the far window," Christine said pointing toward the table. I could see a few friends already gathered.

"Wendy, why don't you head over to the table with Jane and I'll get us a drink," Kim suggested.

"Yes, Wendy, follow me," Jane insisted.

It was not an easy task, the tables were an obstacle every way I looked, but Jane moved chairs out of the way as we progressed toward the rest of the gang. They were all up and moving chairs to clear my path.

"Well hello there stranger," I heard from the distance. It was Don, and with him Gino and Peter.

I was immediately taken aback by the small crowd of friends that had already arrived. I had not been expecting so many to be joining us.

"Well hello to you all," I said back. "I had no idea I would see you here tonight."

"Did you think we would miss your welcome home gathering? It's been too long, Wendy." Gino was sincere in his approach. He had been to Toronto Western Hospital to see me but that was some time ago now.

"How time flies," I responded. "It's so good to see you again."

We moved over to the table as more of the group began to pile in to the bar. To my surprise, the night turned out to be a homecoming celebration planned by my sister and Christine.

"I see your intentions now, Kim. It would appear there are more than a few of my friends gathered here tonight, a very nice gesture. I'm not sure how easy it will be to get around here shortly."

I was thrilled to see everyone again; most of them had been to see me at the hospital. It was hard to believe I was really home and able to be part of the group again. While things were initially accommodating, the bar began to fill up quickly with little room for me, or my wheelchair, to make my way around the tables. Most people attending the celebration came over to me at my table.

Gino was a very close friend to Don, he finally made his way over to me not long after I placed myself at the table they had reserved.

"Hey there, Wendy. What can I say other than how great it is to see you home. You must be happy to have your hospital days behind you."

"Oh yes, more than happy to finally be out of Lyndhurst, although it did serve an incredible purpose, something I would never have anticipated before going there. But it's served me well."

"In what way, Wendy?"

"I guess it has a lot to do with the exposure it gave me to the lives of others who have been through a spinal cord injury, the variables often involved and how grateful I now feel given what I've been exposed to. Things can always be worse. It's by remembering that fact that my life feels worthy of continuing on. We never know what's in store, but we must try our best to overcome the hurdles."

As the night progressed I was entertained by many friends who came over to see me. There must have been 25 people who showed up to wish me well, many of them buying drinks for me. Of course, it was not long before I needed to use the washroom. Kim was informed of this and she came over to me.

"Hey Wendy, it's quite crowded in here now but I'll lead the way," Kim announced, while moving away chairs that were surrounding the table. Many had gone to the dance floor leaving a lot of the chairs unattended. With everyone now scattered throughout the bar the task of making it to the washroom was daunting.

"Come on Wendy, follow me," Kim demanded. The music was now at a high pitch and I could hardly hear her.

"Yes, you lead the way," I responded, dreading the chore of getting there.

We weaved in and out of the crowds with any success only minor with each push of my wheelchair. There were people everywhere and with the music so loud, few of them could hear our pleas to let us through. Ever so slowly we continued through the people, until finally we made it into the washroom facility, only to be met with a lineup of women waiting to use the facilities. My situation really hit home at this time. While there were a number of stalls available, I could only use the one stall modified for my wheelchair, the larger stall found in most public washrooms today. Never would I have thought in all the time seeing those stalls that I would one day rely on them. I was generously offered the stall when it came free by one of the patrons next in line. I made my way into the stall and quickly used the facility. Finally back at the table, I felt tired, frustrated, almost defeated in my efforts. The music was very loud by now, the crowd was larger, and I just wanted to go home. I called my sister over to the table.

"Kim, it's been a long day for me, do you think we could go home now?" I asked.

"Yes, yes of course we could leave, if that's what you want," I could tell Kim knew that I was a little uncomfortable with getting to the washroom through the crowd. We decided we would order some wings and fries before leaving for home.

It was while heading back from the washroom that I had fully realized one of the challenges I was going to face on my journey back into mainstream society. As we were weaving our way through the crowd, I had overheard a girl say to her friend, "Why would *she* come here?" It was not only the logistics of moving around in a wheelchair I would have to overcome. It was also the limiting attitudes of the people around me.

Chapter 10: Introduction to Star Tracks

At first, deciding what to do with my life after returning home from rehab seemed simple enough. Before the accident I had been promoted at Domtar, and they had offered me my old job back, working in the construction division as head of their Arborite product sales. However a visit to the office one day revealed physical obstacles that would make returning to my job a difficult transition. There was a steep incline from the parking lot to the building, impossible for a wheelchair to master alone. There was the entry into the building itself; finally, the filing cabinets that held all the accounts I managed were unreachable from my wheelchair.

Moreover, the reunion with my co-workers was awkward. I felt somewhat helpless, not the woman in complete control as I had been when I'd left the office on the Friday before the accident. The environment I had once ruled with confidence now controlled me. I could not get past what seemed like pity from those colleagues I met that day and I saw that my limitations were now an obvious distraction. I felt by wiping my slate clean and finding new beginnings, there would be no comparisons made to life before losing my mobility, and therefore less to mourn the loss of.

While I was grateful for the offer to return to Domtar, I decided that post-secondary education would be the wisest and most practical choice for me after my injury. I researched entry requirements into both college and university and decided college would be the more practical choice, since I had worked in the real world prior to the accident. I enrolled in Sheridan College's Business Administration course as a full-time student a year and a half following the accident.

I was listening to the radio one morning while getting ready for class when I heard about Star Tracks Talent. The founder, Rhona Mickelson, was being interviewed about starting the agency and what she hoped to achieve.

Unlike most talent agencies, Star Tracks specialized in physically challenged talent. All of Rhona's clients were in wheelchairs, and it was her hope to integrate the disabled into the world of advertising through magazines, catalogues, and flyers. She hoped by offering physically challenged talent, advertisers would eventually use people in wheelchairs in their advertisements.

She was right: We do shop; in fact we do most everything that the able-bodied population does, just a little differently. Our physical challenge does not stop us from living, it just offers more challenging ways to achieve what we want in life.

I wrote the telephone number down when Rhona mentioned it and called it immediately after the interview was over, leaving a message for her to call me back. I figured I had nothing to lose and everything to gain. I had done some modelling in my younger years through the Judy Welch Modelling Agency, and I had done some runway work, but my teeth needed dental work and therefore I had to put things on hold. I wore braces throughout most of high school.

After making the call to Star Tracks, I was ready to hit the road to school.

Returning to college as an adult student put me in a much better frame of mind where my studies were concerned, taking my commitment seriously. I was one of the oldest students in my classes, with honours to my credit as a result of the hard work I put in.

Enrolled in the Business Administration program, with practical business experience behind me through my work at Domtar Construction, I felt I was a great fit with the curriculum. The real benefit was that many of my course instructors were former corporate CEOs; in many ways I could relate to them. I had formal office training in my background and my job at Domtar had included dealing with large corporations.

It is often the practice of Canadian colleges to hire individuals who have worked in the field of study they teach, to give students more of a "first-hand view" of the subject. Often they are able to provide practical examples of what they experienced while working in the field, making the curriculum much more meaningful. I had a high degree of respect for all of my instructors.

The day I heard about Star Tracks on the radio, I arrived at school early for my first class. I was usually there with plenty of time to spare. Today I would only have one morning class, with the rest of the day open for independent study, which I would usually do at home.

The class was Economics, a topic often discussed at the family dinner table, as my father was very politically driven. Fred Dixon, the instructor, reminded me of my great uncle, Mac McDonald. Fred stood tall, had a thin build, with electric blue eyes that captivated you when you met his gaze. He was younger than my Uncle Mac, although old enough to have retired from his corporate position with TD Bank. I loved the course almost as much as I loved Uncle Mac. It was interesting to learn how the economy worked, its fluctuations and what generally caused them. It was the supply and demand theory that really had me captivated, which is the guide to most markets. When demand is high, supply will follow and eventually level the cost in price; when supply is low, then the price is high. Balance is always what you are looking for, if you want markets to be fair.

"Good morning, Wendy," said Fred Dixon as I entered the classroom.

"And a very good morning to you!" was my response.

There were a few students already at their seats. Economics was not a class enjoyed by many of the students and the attendance was often poor. I sat at the front of most classes with my attention well focused on the instructors, to ensure I fully understood what was being taught and to take proper notes for tests and assignments.

"It would seem there are a number of students not attending this morning's class," said Fred. "I wonder if any of you would object to cancelling it, although I do have an assignment for you all to take home. I will leave it up to you all whether you tell the others about this take-home project. Those of you here have an advantage for attending class on time this morning."

We all quickly agreed to the terms while Fred handed printouts of the work to be completed at home. Whether or not to tell the others in class became a big question to us all. While they had missed the early morning class, did that justify them losing out on the marks completing the assignment would bring?

Very few students took the classes as seriously as I did; having been out of school for some time, many of them lacked discipline. I was now better focused than I had been in high school, and I was determined to do well. Getting a good grasp of what was being taught was half the battle. It was then much easier to reacquaint myself with the topics at the time of a test. If what was covered in class made little sense, you could bet studying for the tests and completing assignments would be that much more difficult. I found taking things in stages really worked, and that meant breaking down the lessons one by one.

After class was cancelled I decided to go home to get a head start on the bonus assignment.

After heading into my bedroom and checking my voice mail I noticed I had a message waiting from Rhona Mickelson, requesting that I call her back.

The telephone rang at least three times before I heard a voice on the other end of the receiver.

"Rhona Mickelson here."

"Hello Rhona, Wendy Murphy returning your message. I heard you this morning on CHUM FM and was thrilled to hear you have an agency I would like to become part of."

"Well Wendy, I'm pleased to hear your enthusiasm. Why don't you tell me a little more about yourself and why you feel you would be a good fit for Star Tracks Talent?"

"Well, I was in a car accident that has put me in the wheelchair, and there are a lot of changes I would like to see happen as far as access and exposure are concerned. I do see change coming; however it is not as fast as I had hoped, or in ways I think would really make a difference. Advertising has got to change to reflect the number of people in wheelchairs, all of whom shop for products. Does this make any sense at all?" I asked.

I was hoping my words would resonate with Rhona. There was something missing as far as inclusion in society went; wheelchairs were never seen in advertisements or public notices, although we did exist. It was my hope to change all of that, and perhaps Star Tracks Talent would be my vehicle to do it.

"Wendy, I've been confined to a wheelchair since infancy and certainly relate to the change you are hoping to see happen. People in wheelchairs are definitely more common in the world than we see in advertising. My clients vary in age and disability, but have definitely grown in numbers since I began the business. I have been witness to a number of welcome changes, although I don't believe we're as far as we could be. Let's take this one step at a time. Right now I'd like you to forward me a few photographs, some that best represent you, and we will take it from there."

After we hung up, I realized that the challenge was to find pictures that best represented me, to give Rhona a good idea of just what I looked like.

I made my way into the family room, where my sister was fussing with the blinds, to fill her in on my plan to try and make a difference by going public.

"Well Wendy, you're home early from school."

"Fred Dixon's Economics class was cancelled. Not many showed up and he was upset at the lack of attendance. He offered those of us that did make it a bonus assignment, and you can bet the material handed out today will be on the next test. Putting that aside, I've been in touch with a talent agent, and I plan on sending in a few photos of myself. She's asked for pictures that best represent me.

"I know you have seen the awkwardness I sometimes face when I'm out in public because of the reactions I get to my disability. I'm hoping to change all of that by putting myself and my disability front and centre to show the abilities we have, and to somehow help others to see beyond the disability. There will be attitudes, but if I put my best foot forward, maybe there will be a change in those attitudes. Life is what you make it, and we're here to act on the possibilities. I really feel good about this, and I believe my timing could not be better. I know there will be challenges, but that's been my life since the accident."

"Let's not forget access, Wendy," my sister said, "and the difficulties you might face getting to those meet-and-greet auditions. I'm not here to burst your bubble but I do see difficulties. This is something you will have to work out with the talent agent."

"I'll be sure to bring that up with her. I know I have mentioned wanting to model again in the past but now I feel that this is something that could really happen if Rhona puts me on her roster."

"I see a determined sister who can do just about anything she puts her mind to – she's proven that in the past. Wendy, if it is something you truly want to do, I say go for it."

"We'll be starting with the photographs," I reminded her.

"Yes, that's right. I'll help you choose a few pictures you can send off. You are very photogenic, so I don't see this as a difficult task. Mom is in the kitchen and she can help too."

I wheeled my way through the main floor, into the elevator, and down to the basement where the old chest that stored all our family photographs was kept. Dusting off the frame of the old oak trunk, I dug through the photographs like a scavenger. There were many pictures stored there, giving me a variety of options. Did I want school photographs that showcased my more serious side? Or did the family photographs taken on the beach in Cavendish show me off best? Choosing the right ones to show to my sister and mother was not an easy task.

Unexpectedly, I came upon a collection of photographs that were taken of Grania and me fooling around in our backyard, in our last year of high school. Grania wore a baseball cap and I, an Edmonton Oilers jersey. We both looked so happy and carefree. It brought me back to the time prior to the accident.

I remembered the day well. We had spent the majority of the day in my backyard soaking up the sun and hosing ourselves down when the heat became unbearable.

I took pride in my tan lines and Grania took pride in her ivory skin, which proved to be delicate when overexposed to the sun. She wore a high sunblock tanning lotion to ensure proper protection. I, on the other hand, lived for the sun-kissed brown tone of skin only to be gained while wearing a lower SPF lotion, if any at all. Both Grania and I lived for the finer times in life, and with high school almost over our futures definitely looked brighter and the possibilities endless. What would we do after high school? Where would our relationships go with our boyfriends? What new excitement and experiences would that summer bring?

Storing away the memory, I returned to my task, with pictures now strewn everywhere. I hoped I had a collection of options that would prove worthy for Rhona Mickelson. Was this feasible? I wondered. I had always believed that exposing the issue on a wider scale would bring to light the physically challenged as a functional group of people who somehow found themselves confined to a wheelchair. The limitations many of us were facing were imposed on us through misfortune. Perhaps together, Rhona and I could make a difference that would see the existing attitudes change.

I headed back to the elevator and up to the kitchen, where I found both my mom and sister enjoying a fresh cup of coffee.

"Well Mom, not sure if Kim has filled you in but I am on my way to making changes in my life, and hopefully, to society as a whole."

"What are you up to now?"

"I've been in touch with a talent agent and if all goes well, I'll be represented for modelling jobs for some of the larger department stores here in Canada. The agent has asked that I send her a few photographs and said we would take it from there. I've been down to the chest of drawers and collected a few photos I've got here."

"You're a very photogenic, young lady. I don't see why you wouldn't be accepted into the agency."

I wheeled myself over to join both Kim and my mother at the kitchen table and we sorted through the photographs. Most pictures were of me alone and gave a good sense of my overall size. Most were from before the accident, when I was still walking, but there were photographs with me in the wheelchair as well.

I was never one who really liked getting my photograph taken, often throwing myself into the background when someone took a picture. Now that would all change; I would be presenting myself as a representative of the disabled community, a cause I truly believed in.

It did not take long before we had chosen four pictures showing me in various styles of clothing, one casual and another more formal, taken at my cousin's graduation. We also added two photographs of me wearing a bikini, taken the weekend of the accident. It was the last real memory of me living fully mobile, and it brought on a sense of nostalgia. What once was, was now no longer. I would begin a new journey now. It would be my quest to see change happen within the realm of a society often quick to judge on first impressions and appearances. A society I had once belonged in.

I mailed the photographs out later that evening, with the hope of hearing back from Rhona Mickelson. Star Tracks Talent could prove to be my venue into a more public life, with a justifiable cause behind my efforts.

***

Later that week, Rhona called to say that she loved my photographs, and we set up a meeting at a coffee shop near both our homes.

There was a lot going through my mind as I drove to the meeting. How would the public respond if I signed on with Rhona as a client? How would industry advertisers react to our efforts? I personally saw it as a win-win situation. While the physically challenged community might be less visible, we did exist. Not only would companies benefit by offering a more inclusive role for wheelchairs in advertising their business and products, but they would win the loyalty of consumers actually using wheelchairs.

It was a thirty-minute drive to the coffee shop. Rhona had an advantage: she had my photographs and was able to identify me, so she made the first contact.

She was petite, with long flowing wavy brown hair. She almost appeared lost in her wheelchair. She was dressed in a red maxi skirt and white peasant blouse with a red ribbon that tied around the neck of the garment, giving her outfit a tailored look.

I was upbeat in my initial greeting.

"Hello, and nice to finally meet you, Rhona," I began. "I can't tell you how excited I am to move forward with this."

"Well Wendy, as I mentioned on the telephone, the photographs you sent are very flattering and if my eye tells me anything, you could do very well in this industry."

"Do you really think so?" I asked.

"We're still new in the game but I am hoping to see the larger corporations ready for something different, a more inclusive form of advertising. So far they've been receptive, and I see this as a great time for change. The majority of my clients now are younger – toddlers to twelve years old – and I've received positive feedback from the leaders in advertising."

I was excited to hear that she could actually get work from established outlets like Eaton's and The Bay department stores. Suddenly, I could see no limits as far as where this could go. If advertisers decided to use us in their ads, my mission appeared more attainable: to let wheelchairs be seen in an everyday format and eliminate the public reaction often associated to those who use wheelchairs – the misconceptions and limitations I had often fallen victim to since the accident had occurred.

"I am thrilled to hear your agency is making headway in the advertising industry. I hope in time this will simply be a normal way for advertisers to deliver their messages."

"The progress is there. They are using my clients."

"I see no difference in any of us, however abled we are," I said. "We are consumers, and therefore it only makes sense that we be included in today's markets. I suppose, as a minority, we are facing what many minorities faced in the past. This is now our time for change."

"What I can tell you," said Rhona, "is that many of the companies I have approached have an open mind to using my talent. These are baby steps, but every door that opens brings us one step closer to a more accepting society, one that is more reflective of what truly makes up our communities. Like most things, it takes the innovators to introduce something new, but generally speaking, the competition soon follows."

"Rhona, I look forward to working with you and Star Tracks Talent Agency and bringing about change where the disabled community is concerned. There's no better way to publicly display the fact that we do exist than advertising."

I was quick to sign the contract with Star Tracks Talent Agency. I felt excited to think that I might have the opportunity to go public in my wheelchair through corporate advertising. I was confident that by exposing the issue in advertisements, those of us in wheelchairs would gain more overall acceptance.

The drive home took longer than usual due to a collision. The road was blocked off with ambulances and police everywhere. Seeing the accident at the side of the road gave me time to reflect on my life, the situations I had overcome, and where I found myself today. There was a great deal of loss in and around my own accident; it had put my life initially in such disarray, but with time and patience I was able to move forward and see the many positives that remained. Of course, it also brought a sense of remorse, given Grania was no longer in my life, which intensified all the trials I was forced to face without her. I was riddled with guilt that I had survived the accident and she hadn't. Not only had I survived but I was now living independently. I was attending college and doing well in my classes, and now I had signed a modelling contract with opportunities up to bring my disability to the forefront. I had an opportunity to make a difference for all those finding themselves confined to a wheelchair, regardless of what had put them there, or at what level of physical independence they functioned.

While I took this brief time to reflect, I decided guilt and worry would get me nowhere. Grania would be happy for how my life was going. While I had suffered a great amount of loss, there were positive aspects that could, and would, be my motivation and the focus of my attention now.

Chapter 11: The Bay Shoot

Rhona was tireless in her search for some credible work and showed diligence in her efforts to find me a spot somewhere – anywhere – that would prove advertisers were ready for change.

Her first call came one morning when I was preparing for an exam in Small Business Management. It was obvious from her voice that she was beside herself with excitement.

"Wendy, I hope you are ready for this," she began. "I just received a call from Mary Jo McCoy, stylist for The Bay and she has asked for you! She has a shoot she would like you to be a part of and I am hoping you can make it!"

"The Bay wants me? That's fabulous news! When and where is all of this to take place?"

"Well, their studios are in the northwest end of the city but I am not sure if this shoot will be in the studio or on location."

"On location?"

"You see, Wendy, often the stylists will take a shoot outside of the studio, on location. It might be a park or a restaurant, somewhere that offers a relaxed atmosphere that will enhance the product they hope to advertise."

This sounded like an interesting concept. I understood what she meant about location shooting from the magazines I had read.

"I am thrilled to hear they want to work with me!"

"I am also pleased to see them asking for you," said Rhona. "You are the first adult they've asked for on my roster of clients. I told you those portfolio pictures you had done were impressive. Just look at the work you're getting, and they were only recently sent out. I bet this is just the beginning of something wonderful for you my dear."

I was very pleased to know the pictures appeared to be paying off. The photo shoot had been a full afternoon with Nick Seiflow, one of Toronto's premier photographers for portfolio work. I was there for headshot photographs.

Headshots – eight-by-ten photographs – are used by all the agencies to sell their talent to potential clients. The photos display your features from the shoulders up and what they show can affect the amount and type of work that you get. Hair, makeup, and lighting are crucial to ensure a professional look, and Nick was definitely worth the hundreds of dollars he charged for a professional sitting. I was thrilled with what we ended up with. Having a call come in from The Bay's stylist only confirmed my choice in photographers. You are only as good as your last photo when it comes to the modelling world, and again, Nick Seiflow proved a winner in this case.

"Rhona, I am flexible. I will go where they want me to go."

"I'm glad to hear that. I will let you know the details as I receive them, Wendy."

Thrilled to receive a call for work, I found it difficult to get back into studying. I made my way downstairs to the family room where I found my mother folding laundry.

"Well Mom, you will never guess the news I have to share with you. I received a call from Rhona Mickelson. She sent out the photographs I had done and it appears The Bay would like to include me in their next photo shoot. I don't have all the details yet, but I am thrilled to hear I'm getting work."

"Wendy, that's marvellous news. I knew those photographs would find you work. They're incredible. You must be proud of yourself. You found a photographer, booked for hair and makeup to be done professionally, and now look where you are. I was confident *something* good would come of your efforts."

"Thanks, Mom, although nothing's been confirmed. Rhona said she would contact me when she knows more about the details. I just can't believe this is happening. I am actually going to appear in a Bay catalogue."

"It is your determination I have always believed in. You have always been driven, with your own sense of what is right for you. Nothing you do could surprise me. I have seen you accomplish so much over the years. When you put your mind toward doing something, you are fearless."

"I suppose I can become pretty determined in my pursuits," I agreed. "It comes naturally for me to want to follow through on my plans, and I guess that has been what has driven me over the years. You and Dad deserve some of the credit. You have both always supported me on any goals I've hoped to achieve."

With the conversation reflective in nature, I suddenly felt the loss of Grania and thought how she would add to my excitement. She was always supportive of my endeavours and this news would prove no exception. I knew that she would be there to cheer me on in my hope and determination to make a difference publicly for wheelchairs.

"This has been a difficult week for me. While I am excited to see things evolve, I can't help but miss Grania. I know she would be thrilled to see this happen and support me through it all. There are moments I feel I am taking too much on, while on the other hand, I feel it's time for me to do this now. I'm sometimes torn."

"There is no reason to feel torn, Wendy. You are moving forward in a very positive direction. The universe appears to be in your favour right now. Grania has left a remarkable void in your life, and there's no doubt about the loss you must feel at certain times. That loss can now be turned into incredible memories. She lives on within you, her spirit will keep you going. Keep her close to your heart."

"What a beautiful way to see it," I responded. "And you are right. She does live on in my memory, and she will always remain close to my heart."

On that note, I excused myself from the conversation to make my way back to my room. My Small Business Management test would be in the coming week, and I did hope to do well on it.

Studying was not something I thoroughly enjoyed; however, I had set high standards for myself where grades were concerned. Only through studying would I see those marks, and therefore getting back to the books was important.

Shortly after I entered the room, the telephone rang. It was Rhona.

"Hi Wendy, I have heard from Mary Jo and have all the details for you regarding the photo shoot. It's scheduled to take place tomorrow. I am hoping you are still game for the job."

"Yes, yes of course I am still game. What are the details?"

"Well, the shoot will take place in studio, so there will be no worries finding your way through the big city of Toronto. They are located at 2595 Summerhill Drive and the studio is fully accessible. Your hair and makeup will be done for you, so go with basic hair preparation and no makeup. I believe you will be modelling a pair of Levi's jeans. What you will need to bring are some shoes that you would wear with blue jeans, the rest will be supplied. Does all of this make sense to you?"

"Not sure exactly where the studio is located but I'll look it up in my Perly's Map Book. Things are easy if I don't have to prepare for the shoot. I can certainly supply the shoes."

"It is scheduled to take place at 11:30 a.m. I am hoping this will work for you. Give yourself plenty of time to find the studio, as you wouldn't want to be late."

"Tomorrow will definitely work for me. In fact, I am really looking forward to it! I already have three pairs of shoes in mind to bring along with me. Is there someone I should ask for?"

"Oh yes, it will be Mary Jo, the stylist. She is really looking forward to meeting you. She was very impressed with your photographs," Rhona added.

"I am thrilled to be a part of this. I cannot wait to meet her!"

Thrilled to hear the job was mine, I made my way throughout the house to be sure that all family members were aware of my news. I found my sister Kim in the front hallway, preparing to go out.

"Kim, Kim you'll never guess what is happening! I can hardly believe it myself! I had a telephone call from Rhona Mickelson and I'm booked to do a photo shoot with The Bay. Can you believe it? They want me!"

"That is fabulous news, Wendy, but I don't have a lot of time to talk. I'm just on my way out to an appointment. Can we take things up where we left off when I get back?"

"I guess we could, if you have no time right now. I will have to bring my own shoes for the shoot and I already have a few pairs in mind. I thought the camel flats would work, as well as the black heels, and—"

"Wendy, I really have no time right now. I promise when I get back...."

She ran out the door before finishing her sentence.

With Kim fleeing my good news and no one left to share it with, I decided studying would be my best bet. Small Business Management was a class I did well in and maintaining my average was a priority. I went back to my room and gathered the shoes I planned to bring to the photo shoot the following morning. Then I remained cocooned for hours, surrounded by study sheets and books, until I was called to the dinner table by my mother.

I could not wait to share the exciting news with my father and my brother, Jeff.

"Well, have you both heard the exciting news?" I asked.

"What news?" my brother responded.

"You are looking at a woman who will grace the pages of the soon-to-be-created Hudson Bay flyer. I received a call from Rhona Mickelson earlier today asking if I would be available for a shoot to take place at their studio tomorrow morning. Those photographs I had done by Nick Seiflow have really paid off. I am apparently the first adult model they have asked for and I am busting at the seams to know this is actually going to happen!"

"That is really great news," my father responded. "Where will all of this take place?"

"The studio is in the east end of the city. I have little responsibility other than getting myself there on time with a few pairs of shoes to wear for the shoot. I will be modelling Levi's jeans."

"Wow sis, that's pretty exciting!" said my brother. "Will you be getting the model treatment, hair and makeup done by the professionals?"

"Yes, all the preparations will be done for me. I was told to arrive with clean hair and no makeup, making the day as easy as pie. My only real task is to be there on time. Since this is my first professional job I am a little nervous. I wonder about the others and their reaction to seeing me there for the shoot. I know I am the first older model in a wheelchair they have selected to be part of the flyer and catalogue for their customers. I'm just not sure of the reaction I'll be facing when I actually get to the studio."

"This is something you have hoped to achieve for some time now Wendy," said my father. "I hope you won't dwell too much on what others might think or say. It's obvious those responsible for hiring the talent for this job see that you are competent. That's all that should be important to you right now."

I knew what he was saying was true, but for me there was always self-doubt when it came to meeting anyone since the accident. I often felt there was something to prove, and I did my best to have others see me and not the wheelchair. I did not want to be measured by the limitations others placed on me.

"You are right, Dad, and I know how you all see it. But until you've walked a mile in my shoes, you can't speak from my experience. There are definitely people who do not initially see beyond my wheelchair, and I face them on a daily basis. They see my limitations as much greater than they really are and often feel uncomfortable with something as simple as conversation with me. I don't know if they imagine my life to be limited as a result of my challenges. They don't see all that I'm now involved in. I drive my own car, I'm a full-time student, and I get out with friends on a regular basis. There is little lacking in my life, and others don't always see the full picture. I often feel pegged with sympathy when I meet strangers out in public, and that usually becomes more obvious by their statements: 'Hello dear, is there something I can help you with? You look like you could use some help.' Somehow, it's assumed I'll need assistance. That's just one scenario. I face it almost everywhere I go."

"Then it is up to you to teach those that are unenlightened," replied my father. "You can't go through life feeling overly sensitive when others are merely showing a kind heart. I'm sure they only want to help when they approach you."

"Maybe you are right in some instances, but there are other times I know they see nothing but the wheelchair, which often segregates me. It is my hope to one day live barrier free. The rest of the world often sets limited standards on what can be achieved by those in wheelchairs, and I do not want to be defined by those standards. Can you understand my perspective?"

"I trust that your perspective is clear, but my fear is that you may be subject to the attitudes you believe are limiting you, or in some way categorizing you because of the wheelchair. I would hope that you'd keep an open mind and heart to those who are merely trying to help."

While my father and I had shared a very sensitive topic, my whole family tried to understand where I was coming from. Many of them had experienced the stares and gestures while out with me.

My sister jumped into the conversation to offer the observations she had made.

"I believe the attitudes you often face come from lack of knowledge. Let's not forget where we were as a family immediately after your diagnosis, and how little knowledge we had about what you could accomplish using the wheelchair. I don't believe we all saw you in a progressive way initially. Most people have a lack of insight when it comes to spinal cord injury. We were there once. That usually doesn't change until you are somehow associated with someone who's actually had a spinal cord injury. What you are doing now could have monumental results over time when it comes to changing those attitudes. You've definitely come a long way, little sister!"

It was through this discussion that we were able to come to a better understanding of what I often faced while out in public and what my family members observed when they were out with me.

I went to bed early that night to be sure I was up and ready for the photo shoot. Finding the actual studio would be one of the challenges I faced, as well as the hope of full access for the wheelchair.

Where access was concerned, facing the unknown often became par for the course. While changes were coming around with ramps and accessible washrooms, I could not always be sure that I would find complete access everywhere I went.

Photos

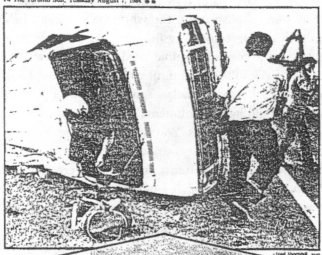

14 The Toronto Sun, Tuesday August 7, 1984

— fred thornhill, sun

WOMAN KILLED AS VAN FLIPS

A tow truck crew prepares to remove a van in which a Mississauga woman was killed and two people were hurt last night when the van rolled over on the ramp from northbound Hwy. 403 to Hwy. 401. OPP said Grania O'Neill, 18, of Manion Rd., died of head injuries and a slashed throat when she was thrown about 50 feet.

Article of actual accident

Picture of Grania

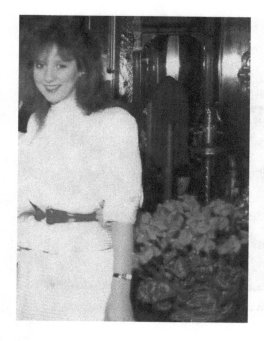

Me with Fiona

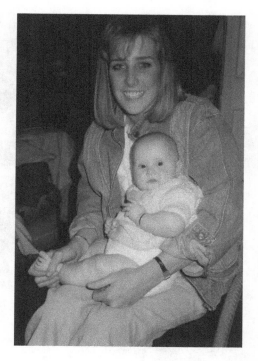

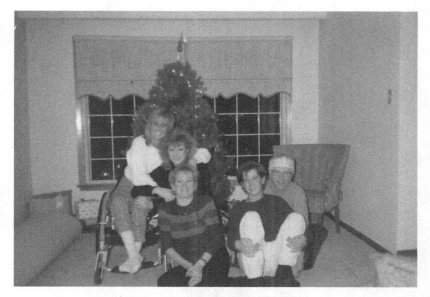

First Christmas in our newly renovated home

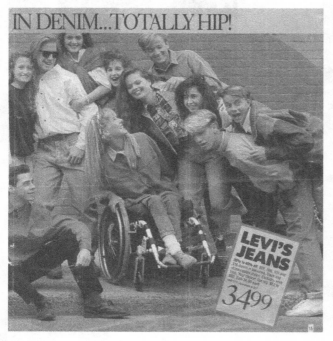

Bay shoot for
Levi's jeans

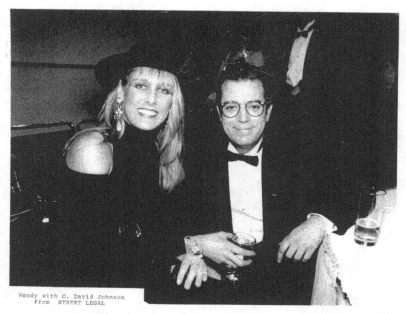

Wendy with C. David Johnson
from STREET LEGAL

Me with C. David Johnson from Street Legal at Gemini Awards

Skiing at Silver Star Ski
Resort; Vernon, British
Columbia

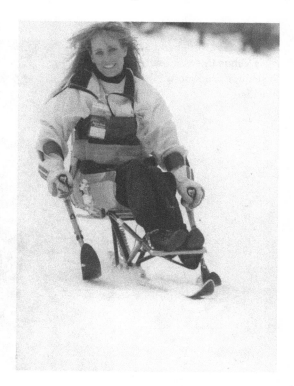

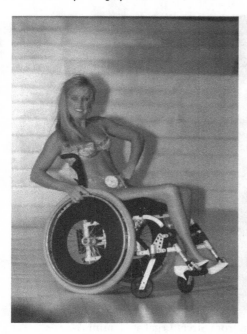

Bikini segment at Miss Venus International Pageant; Boca Raton, Florida

Evening Gown segment at Miss Venus International Pageant; Boca Raton, Florida

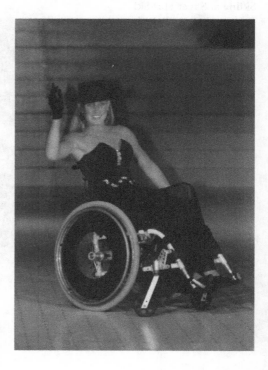

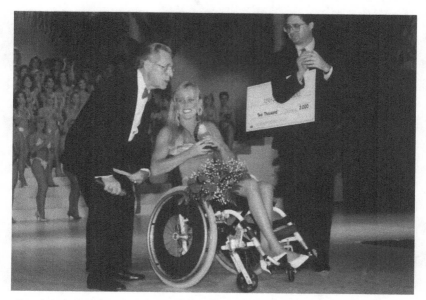

Receiving Contestants Choice Award at Miss Venus International Pageant;
Boca Raton, Florida

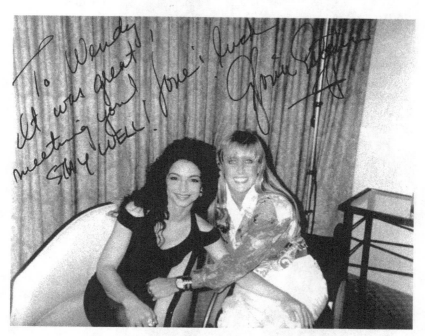

Gloria Estefan and I following interview in Montreal

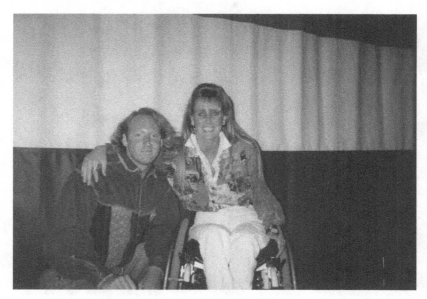

Glen Baxter and I following Gloria Estefan concert in Montreal

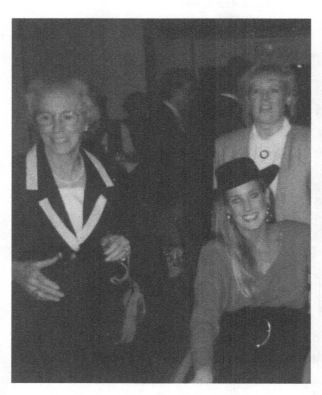

Mother and I with Betty Kennedy at Front Page Challenge reception; Charlottetown, PEI

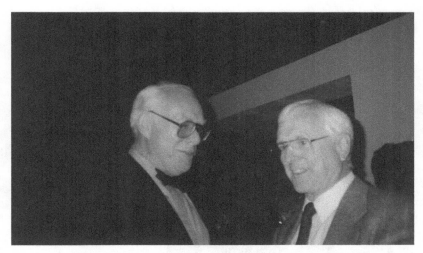

Dad with Pierre Burton at Front Page Challenge reception; Charlottetown, PEI

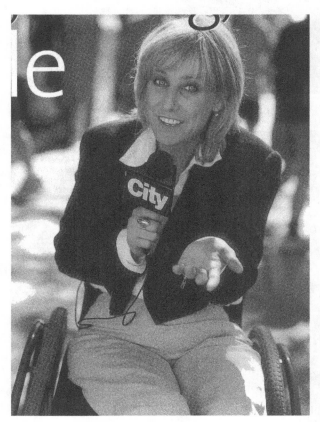

Me reporting for City TV

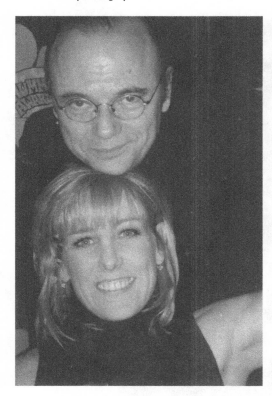

Me with Moses Znaimer
from City TV

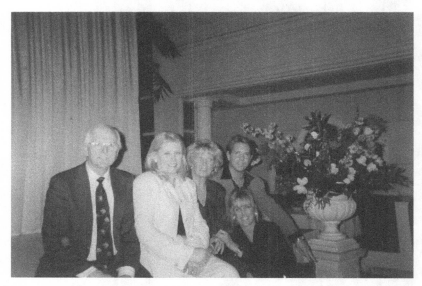

Me with the family at Woman Who Makes a Difference Award ceremony

Chapter 12: Changing Attitudes

Finding my way to the studios was smooth sailing and I was pleased to locate an accessible parking spot; there was also an automatic door opener on the entrance of the building. Things are looking up, I thought, as far as access is concerned.

I introduced myself to the receptionist, who paged Mary Jo to meet me.

The office reception was basic in style and sparse in furniture. I was a little surprised given the studio was there to welcome visitors and encourage the world of fashion. I had been told the majority of The Bay's merchandise was promoted through this studio, and I expected something more from its overall look.

In a few moments, Mary Jo appeared.

"Hello Wendy. It's a pleasure to finally meet you. Did you find us all right?" she asked.

"It's a pleasure to finally meet you as well, Mary Jo. I had no trouble at all finding you here this morning."

Mary Jo was middle aged, with a medium build and blonde hair. She was very stylish in her appearance and stood about five feet eight inches tall. She wore a three-quarter length pant with a loose blouse and wedged heel. She was an attractive woman, with a pleasant demeanour, looking ready to jump in front of the camera herself.

"Let's get you into the change room and start your hair and makeup. I have chosen a few outfits for you to model."

We followed a long corridor that took the form of a maze as we made our way into the back change room. There were already two girls sitting in the hair and makeup chairs.

"Hello to you all," I announced as I wheeled into the room. "My name is Wendy and this is my first time participating in the modelling shoot so I'd welcome any insights. Have you both been here before?"

Both models began to answer at the same time.

"Yes, I've been here before and I have worked with Mary Jo on many occasions inside the studio. My name is Kara."

"My name is Liz, and I've been here at the studio many times. In fact, I believe they've designated a parking spot for me! What agency are you with Wendy?"

"My agency is Star Tracks Talent. It's relatively new and specializes in physically challenged talent. I guess my agent saw a niche that had yet to be filled and developed her business with that concept in mind."

"Interesting idea," Liz replied.

"Enough of the chatting girls, there is work to be done here," were Mary Jo's words. "There'll be time for socializing when we get these photos finished. Wendy, I believe Carol is ready for you."

I moved over to Carol, the makeup artist, to begin the process. Both hair and makeup took close to an hour and I was certainly a sight by the end of both procedures. My eyes had never looked so blue and my hair was full, much like what you would see in the magazines. They added hot rollers and close to a can of hairspray, which gave my hair the full-on treatment, and a more polished effect to the overall look. I had often wondered how those women in magazines looked so well presented. I now had a better idea.

Shortly after my hair and makeup were completed, Mary Jo entered the room with some clothes on hangers and presented both Liz and me with a few each.

"You can both begin with these outfits," she instructed.

They were Levi's jeans, just as Rhona had said. The mock neck jersey Mary Jo handed to me was navy and Liz was passed the same jersey in a taupe colour. Mary Jo went on to explain that we would be doing a photo shoot together, both wearing the Levi jeans and a mock neck jersey. We made our way into the individual change rooms and came out looking very similar in style, although Liz had brown hair, cut in a traditional bob style, with me blonde and my hair at more of a medium length. Liz stood a towering five foot eleven and commanded the room with her presence.

"Now both of you follow me and I'll introduce you to Marshall, who will be your photographer today."

Mary Jo sounded pleased with the look we both shared as we all made our way into the studio. It was a mainly dark but spacious room with a white screen pulled down from the ceiling and covering a good portion of the floor. The camera tripod was set up in front of the white screen, and Marshall was beside it. He stood an average height with a heavy build – he looked at least fifty pounds overweight. Not what I would expect for a fashion photographer. He certainly could clean up his act in a number of ways, I thought: clothes and hair to start. I supposed he was not the one going before the camera lens. He was there to shoot the photographs.

"Hello girls, and welcome," were Marshall's initial words of encouragement. "Well Mary Jo, it appears we have a newcomer with us today."

His words made me feel somewhat awkward and unattached, as if I was singled out from the threesome we had seemed to establish while in hair and makeup. I was well acquainted to both Liz and Mary Jo by now and feeling comfortable in my own skin. The wheelchair no longer seemed an issue between us. This would now change, and getting comfortable with my circumstances seemed appropriate since Marshall was now part of the group.

"Yes Marshall, meet Wendy. This is her first photo shoot for The Bay, and Liz and I have been prepping her on the job," Mary Jo responded.

"Wendy, it's a pleasure to meet you, and not to worry, I've worked with a great many number of newbies. I'll walk you through this like you've been doing it all your life."

"Hello Marshall, the pleasure is all mine," I replied. "I'm relieved to know that you have my back here. I am a quick learner."

Everyone began to laugh with the banter back and forth. Suddenly it was as though Marshall and I had known each other all along, sharing jokes and conversing. I did my best to remain comfortable, although still I felt very anxious and uncomfortable with it all. Being in a wheelchair and modelling clothing put a much different spin on what the fashion industry is all about: it seeks perfection. I was far from perfect, and in so many ways.

Mary Jo stepped in to get us all set up and prepared for the first roll of film. She threw me a scarf to put around my neck and passed Liz a jean vest to swing over her shoulder. There was music playing in the back ground and Marshall began coaching us from behind his camera lens.

"Okay girls give me a nice big smile, thaaat's it.... Wendy, lean in a little to your left, closer to Liz, and Liz you gesture to Wendy as though you're pointing to something out in the distance."

It was all remarkably clever, and made sense. That's how those catalogue photographs look so natural, I thought. They always appear to be having such a good time in them. Now I knew the secret. I had often marvelled over the pictures in the advertisements I would see in catalogues and magazines. It had always seemed that everyone was in a place I would rather be, whether the ad was selling clothing or toothpaste. The individuals in the ads were always so animated and seemed to be having the time of their lives. I knew now this was all part of the job. Expressions and gestures were encouraged by the models job to bring in readers, to clinch the sale.

Mary Jo came into the screened area every now and then to fix our clothes, hair, or add another prop or piece of clothing. Almost two full rolls of film were used in the first session, and then we were ushered back to the change room to change into our second outfits. It was then that I was able to share all my thoughts and impressions to both Mary Jo and Liz, and there was so much going through my mind.

"Wow, was that something!" were my initial words. "There is so much to see behind the scenes that I hardly know where to look."

"It's all so normal for me now," Liz replied, "although I do remember feeling as you do now when I first stepped in front of the camera lens for a paying job. There is a lot to learn. I've just lost the initial impression of it all after all the years I have been doing this."

Before I could respond, Mary Jo entered the room to rush the process.

The second photo shoot had me in jogging pants and a sweatshirt. I had not anticipated workout attire and hadn't brought any running shoes with me. After I was fully changed, I returned to the photo studio.

"Well Wendy, I don't see those as an appropriate shoe with what you are modelling in this shoot," Mary Jo said, as I entered the white screen area where the pictures were to be taken.

"Mary Jo, I didn't bring any running shoes along. I wasn't sure what type of shoe would be required, so I brought a few on the dressier side."

"That's not a problem. We'll have Marshall shoot you from just above the knees, with no shoes necessary. That's the creative problem-solving side of me talking now," Mary Jo was quick to add.

The shoot lasted a total of three hours, including hair and makeup. The experience opened my eyes to the world of advertising: the many influences relied upon when trying to sell a product, not to mention the preparation time. It also assured me that my hope of exposing the issue of disability through advertising – the fact that we did exist in productive ways – was not an unattainable goal. I felt that my efforts were finally beginning to pay off, and I knew that it would only be a matter of time before we would find a place and voice within society. Change would come about through an agency like Star Tracks Talent, and I remained certain that it was only a matter of time before the industry would feel the moral obligation to include us in their advertisements. I was pleased that it was beginning with a company as established and renowned as The Hudson's Bay Company, not to mention the encouraging welcome that I was given by Mary Jo. Having her on board would be more of an indication that work from The Bay just might continue.

I found the work, and possibilities for more work, very exciting. I could not help but reflect on how far I had come since the accident. Never could I have imagined that I would find such independence again, although the doctors at Toronto Western Hospital had been adamant that I would. They had all anticipated my independence around home, transfers to and from the wheelchair, even driving my own vehicle using hand controls. I had achieved more than most people would have anticipated. I now saw tasks like the modelling job I'd just done as an achievable possibility thanks to my agent, Rhona.

When I got home, she was the first person I shared the experience with by telephone, leaving nothing out.

Chapter 13: Street Legal

With much of my print work circulating through the fashion and modelling industry, Rhona suggested that I begin reading for television work through ACTRA.

ACTRA, the Alliance of Canadian Cinema, Television and Radio Artists, represents professional performers working in English-language recorded media across Canada. The fees were reasonable and the benefits for members included better minimum wages and the oversight of work-related regulations. It is the work permits you receive as a non-union actor that eventually qualify you to join ACTRA. This can be a long, drawn out process, but eventually I became a full member.

One afternoon I received a call from Rhona.

"Wendy, I have some great news. I've received a phone call from CBC casting and they're looking for a courtroom stenographer for the weekly show, Street Legal. Is this something you'd be interested in reading for?"

Not familiar with the process of auditioning, I asked questions.

"Reading for a part is all new to me, Rhona. When did they want me to audition? What's the preparation time like?"

"The audition is this Thursday. It's not a big part, maybe two lines, but it would look great on your résumé. It would also pay at a higher scale now that you are an ACTRA member. This would be a great opportunity for you, Wendy, if you are willing to go for it," Rhona insisted.

Reading for a part was something I had longed to do. The television show Street Legal was a show I watched occasionally. I was thrilled with the opportunity.

"What about the studio where the series is being filmed? Do you know if it's accessible, will I get in with my wheelchair okay?"

"I've made some inquiries and it would seem there are a few stairs at the front of the building. They've assured me that there'll be plenty of crew hands onsite who can help. What do you say, is it something you want to do?"

"I would love to be part of the production. What's the next step?" I asked.

"I'll fax you the script this evening so you can go over it. The address is 900 Dupont Street, and I'll be sure to get you the direct contact number before the audition. I think it's fabulous you've agreed to this, Wendy. If you have any questions, please do not hesitate to call me."

"Thanks, Rhona. This is a great opportunity, let's see where it goes!" I replied.

After our telephone conversation I made my way down to the family room. My good friend, Gina, was on her way over for the evening and there was some tidying up to do around the house before I'd feel prepared to host her. I was greeted by my mother as I entered the room.

"There you are," she said. "I have been in search of someone, anyone, capable of putting this room back in order. Your brother Jeff and his friend Andrea have left it upside down after their video games."

"I'll do my best to put the room back in order. I have Gina coming to visit this evening. It's been a while since I've seen her, so there's lots to catch up on."

The friendship between Gina and me went back to early high school and there were many memories that we shared prior to my accident. Gina had just purchased a new red sports car and wanted to show it off.

We had all wondered if she'd ever bite the bullet and trade in her white Camaro, a car she took pride in driving for more than a decade. It was definitely time for a replacement and I was bursting with anticipation waiting for her to finally arrive. I was making myself useful putting cushions back on the couches and stacking away the video games that were strewn across the floor when my sister Kim entered the room.

"Hey there Wendy. I've definitely seen this room in better order. How can I help? Was Jeff in here with his friends again?"

"You know him too well. Thanks for the help. Gina is on her way over for a visit. She's finally purchased a new car and will be bringing it by to show it off. Not just any car, I might add, a brand new Stealth."

"A Stealth? I've seen the ads for that car, it's quite the vehicle. What are those cars worth anyway?"

"That's not something I know offhand. Gina's the one to be asking. She'll be here any minute."

Shortly after we got the family room organized Gina arrived.

"Hello ladies, nice to see you both," she said.

Kim and I both approached her, arms opened wide; I was trying to wheel while making the gesture. Gina laughed and approached me first.

"That's more like it. How are my girls doing anyway?" she asked while hugging the two of us.

"Doing just fine," we answered in unison. "In fact, I couldn't be better," I continued.

Both Kim and Gina stared at me, knowing from my tone of voice, something was up.

"I received some pretty exciting news from my agent this afternoon. It looks like I'll be reading for a part on the series Street Legal later this week. I'm pretty pumped for this."

"Do tell us more, Wendy," Gina insisted.

"There's not much more to tell really. I received a phone call from Rhona, my agent, who told me CBC was asking for a courtroom stenographer. The part might be all of two lines, but I think I'm going to go for it."

"That's fabulous news. I hope it all works out for you, little sister," Kim added.

Putting my good news aside, we all went out to the front yard to check out Gina's new sports car. And sporty it was. It sat low to the ground with steel belted radial tires. It had a back spoiler, an incredible stereo and a plush interior. We were both impressed. While my sister insisted on a test drive, I declined, knowing the seats were much too low for me to transfer into. I also feared the wheelchair might mark up the car.

The week seemed to breeze by. I was busy getting caught up on school assignments and preparing for some upcoming tests.

Serious about my schooling, I tried to stay ahead of the game with my workload. My intentions were to keep my marks up while pursuing my mission for increased public awareness on disability. I was constantly facing extended stares while out in public with others. People would often speak only to those I was with, as if I wasn't there. This put a strain on my efforts to remain independent, not to mention the frustrations I felt while attempting to move on with my life.

The morning of the CBC audition arrived and I was excited, knowing what was ahead of me, and what might come of it. Having received an audition call from such a large corporation spoke volumes, and both Rhona and I were aware of this. Rhona had sent out endless press releases promoting the agency and we, as a team, had met with a number of reporters in the hope of creating exposure and work for the agency. It now appeared our efforts were paying off.

When I arrived at the studio, I drove into the parking area on the east side of the building. There were a number of people outside the building, who appeared to be on a cigarette break. I approached them, not entirely sure I had reached the right building.

"Good morning," I offered to the group. "My name is Wendy, and I am here to do some work for the Street Legal production. Would any of you know where I should be? Better yet, can I enter okay with the wheelchair?"

They were all sitting on a staircase at the side of the building, which had me worried that stairs getting in to the building might be involved.

"You'll have to go around to the other side of this building, and there will be a few stairs once you get there," said one of the men. "Not to worry though, a couple of us will meet you there and offer you a hand."

I was lost for words and had to take a second look at the handsome gentleman who had offered such a kind gesture. More than that, I had found my way to the proper place, with access not a real issue anymore. I would make it in to my audition thanks to the assistance of some very kind strangers.

After being carried up three steps around the side of the building, I found my way into what appeared to be a set for the production. Not long afterward, I was approached by an older woman who introduced herself.

"Hello, you must be Wendy," she said pleasantly, while extending her hand. I'm so glad you made it into the building all right. My name is Kara Clancey. I am head of casting here."

I was impressed by her formal introduction, but more so by her gesture. She had reached out to shake my hand, resolving any issues I had thought she might have with the wheelchair. There was an immediate form of acceptance. I felt no different from anyone else there to audition for the part, and that feeling came thanks to the generous actions of Kara Clancey.

"Hello Kara. Yes, I am Wendy, and it's my pleasure to meet you," I responded.

"Well Wendy, you're here in plenty of time. One of the casting directors has called with car problems so we're awaiting his arrival. Can I get you a drink while we wait?"

"I'll have some water if that's not too much trouble. And is there a place where I can go over my lines?" I asked.

"Yes, of course. There are two rooms down the hall and to your right."

Arriving at the room, I was surprised to find a group of people, all with scripts in their hands, who were obviously there for an audition. Just what part they were vying for was anyone's guess. I made my way to the right-hand corner, where I sat with at least two others who were busy going over lines.

Soon, my name was called from behind a partially opened door that led into another room.

"Wendy Murphy, we're ready for you. Come in here and have a go at it."

I confidently wheeled past the others seated in the room and through the doorway. I could feel my blood pressure rise briefly when I found myself face to face with four individuals all sitting behind a long banquet-type table. They had water bottles in front of them and sat with what many would consider stone cold expressions on their faces.

"Well, good morning to you all!" I said as I wheeled into the stark white room.

"Good morning," two of them said simultaneously, while the other two took their time.

"Not sure how long you'll all be in here, but you're definitely missing a beautiful day outside," I added.

"Thanks for that, Wendy. We hope to get out there soon," the only woman of the four responded. "Now I believe you know why you're here and your lines are very brief. Can we hear you say them while John reads the lines with you?"

Before I knew it there was a tall gentleman heading toward me with a copy of the script. He stood well over six feet, and he had jet black hair with dark-coloured eyes. His body was to die for.

I took the script from his right hand. "Now John, where would you like me to be for the reading, unless where I'm sitting right now will do?"

I threw them all off. I believe they were taken aback by my forthright manner and confidence. All three sitting behind the table smiled, while John took his place behind me.

"Your line comes following a judge's question about what's been said during the trial, Wendy," John explained.

"The defendant has just responded to the judge's question, and you are reading back her response," explained the woman sitting behind the table.

This gave me a much better understanding of just what was happening in the scene, and a better insight into portraying the character I was auditioning for. I knew the job of a courtroom stenographer, but could I act one appropriately enough?

"'Yes, your honour. As I told the police officers, the front door was fully opened when I approached the home.'"

That was it! My debut as an actor, and I had said the line correctly. Whether it was acceptable to the casting director was now the question. He offered his input.

"That was good, Wendy. I wonder if you could put a longer pause in the sentence. 'As I told the police officers' ... pause ... 'the door was fully opened when I approached the home.' But that was good. I just feel a longer pause would give it more credibility. Please, try again."

I took his advice and repeated the line. This time he seemed to like it. There was little said, other than it was better, and a thank-you for your time. I wondered what the outcome would be, although I was leery as to whether I would hear from them.

"Thank you very much for your time, Wendy. We'll be in touch with your agent," was how the audition ended. More like a *Don't call us, we'll call you* type of dismissal.

I was happy to have it over with, although a little surprised at how quickly the whole event happened. Who knew what would come of the situation now? I would have to await word from Rhona about how well I had done.

I found my way home by reversing the same directions that had brought me there. I was not a daring driver and the highways often intimidated me. I was now driving with hand controls, which put a little more question into the mix where speed and safety were concerned. I had taken the back roads to the audition, directions offered by my father that were sure to get me there safely and on time.

Shortly after arriving home I received a phone call from Rhona.

"Hello Rhona. Have you heard from anyone in the casting department? How did I do?"

"Well Wendy, I have some great news. I did get a call from Kara and it appears they liked what they saw. They were impressed with you, and yes, you've received the part of Jenna the Courtroom Stenographer. Congratulations!"

***

Knowing exactly where I was heading made my drive to the TV studio for the Street Legal episode that much easier. I now knew my route and final destination, thanks to my father and his Perly's Map Book. While driving with the hand controls became second nature after time, I did not need any distractions to sway my concentration. Proper directions made things easier when finding my way on new routes.

I arrived at the building almost an hour earlier than my scheduled arrival time to ensure I would find the same help getting into the building that I had the day of my audition. Would it all go as smoothly as my initial visit?

Looking around, I did not notice anyone outside the building. I used my car phone and the contact number I'd been given to call the studio and let them know I had arrived.

People's reaction to my physical independence had become the norm and at times almost humorous to me. I had grown very self-reliant over time, often amazing myself at how far I had come and the things I could now do on my own.

The wheelchair I would place in the backseat while sitting with my feet outside the car, then tilting the bucket seat forward, which allowed adequate space for the chair to be pulled in and placed, front wheels first, up on the backseat. I took the chair out by reversing the process.

The wheelchair was out of the car and I was lifting myself onto it when three men came from around the back of the building.

I could see by their reaction that they were impressed by my independence in manoeuvering myself out of the car, not to mention the car itself. I was driving a candy-red Firebird, with a license plate that read SASSI. Not what most would imagine someone with paraplegia to be driving, if they were driving at all.

"My name is Blake," said one of the men. "I'm in charge of set preparation. Just tell us what we can do to help you."

We made our way around the building and the three of them assisted me up the few stairs at the other side of the studio. I would need to find hair and makeup. Rhona had told me the director would want to go over the scene before taping began, and I was prepared for that. I felt better that we would have a rehearsal, reducing the chance that I would mess anything up.

After entering the building I was directed to the hair and makeup room by Blake. While making a short turn around a corner I was met by one of the stars of the show, Sonja Smits.

"Well hello there," she said.

"Hello," I said stopping myself from going any further.

"I guess you're looking for hair and makeup. You'll find both rooms straight down the hallway. They'll be on your right-hand side."

I could not believe I was actually right in front of Sonja Smits! Sonja was even more beautiful in person than on TV, with not a blemish on her skin, or hair out of place. She stood about five foot seven, with auburn hair and her dazzling eyes. They smiled as genuinely as she seemed.

She continued down the hall walking in the opposite direction, toward what I knew must be the set, with all the lights, noise, and confusion coming from the area.

Following Sonja's directions I made my way into hair, a room that was also very brightly lit up, with mirrors covering the walls.

"Hi, you must be Jenna, I mean Wendy – you'll be taking on the role of Jenna today. My name is Mary. It's a pleasure to meet you."

I said little as I tried to make my way through the room with four tall chairs in a row. It was obvious the chairs offered better access for Mary to work on hair, with the light illuminating better from the higher level.

"Come in and get settled. Not to worry about the chairs. I'll be fine doing your hair from your wheelchair. It's a basic style they've asked for, an everyday look."

I was relieved to know I wouldn't have to climb into one of the higher chairs.

"Julie from makeup will be coming in to get you all ready with makeup. The makeup room is up a few stairs so we thought it better if she came to you."

Mary moved around my wheelchair and began combing my hair. It was a little past shoulder length at that time, and easy to work with. Just as we were finishing up I heard a male voice coming through the intercom.

"Mary, Ben here. Is Wendy there with you?"

"Yes Ben, she's here."

"We've had a change in shooting plans and are going to move on to Wendy's scene in the courtroom. Is she ready to go?"

"She'll be ready in no time." At that point, a young girl came into the room with a large bag draped over her shoulder with blush brushes sticking out of it.

"Hey Julie," said Mary. "This is Wendy, who'll be playing the role of Jenna in the courtroom today. I just have to add a bit of hair spray … and … here you go."

"Hey Wendy," said Julie. "Sorry for you to have to be rushed this way but what Ben wants as set producer, Ben gets. We'll get through this no problem."

She began rustling through her bag, pulling out foundation and eyeliners. I suddenly felt like an important piece of the puzzle. I could get used to this kind of treatment, I thought.

"You've got some great features to work with, Wendy. Mary, take a look at those blue eyes!"

My eyes were one feature that always garnered attention. They were a gift from my mother's side of the family and are strikingly blue. They are different from my brother's and sister's, much lighter in shade.

Before too long, my makeup was complete and I was ready to go. I did not feel myself, and seldom did after having professional makeup applied. It was always such a heavier look than with the makeup I applied everyday. I looked up to see a young man coming into the room.

"Hey there Wendy, I'm Jason and I'm here to get you to the set. No real rush, they're adjusting the lights. We have time."

Jason was younger, I would guess about nineteen years of age. He was cute, with jet black hair and blue eyes. He took control of the situation.

"Just follow me this way, Wendy. Have you been on a film set before?"

"No Jason. Is there something I should know about?" I joked.

"Heck no," he replied laughing. "I was just curious."

The journey was smooth until we reached the actual set. The lighting cables were everywhere and I had to do wheelies to get over most of them. Jason eventually took over, getting me to where I needed to be. With vaulted ceilings approximately thirty feet high it was an intimidating atmosphere. There were cameras everywhere.

"Welcome Wendy," I heard from across the room. I recognized the voice's owner immediately from the day I auditioned. It was John, the man who had directed me through my audition.

"Glad to see you've made it," he added while walking across the set toward me.

"I made it here fine. I'm thrilled," I added.

I looked around to see if I would see any of the characters I watched on television, but saw no one I recognized.

"I hope they've been treating you well around here."

"With kid gloves," I responded.

"Okay," John yelled out. "We have Jenna on set now. Let's get everyone back here and shoot scene twelve, episode nine while we still have Eric and Sonja!"

I knew he was referring to Eric Peterson and Sonja Smits – Leon and Carrie from the series. I was hoping not to be too star-struck; it was quite a thrill to be up close with them both.

John made his way over to me looking serious.

"Okay Wendy, I want to see you enter the courtroom for this scene by wheeling down the court hallway. Leon and Carrie will be walking toward each other and you'll be wheeling first behind, but then beside, Sonja. They'll stop in front of the courtroom to talk but before they do, you'll wheel past Sonja and in front of Eric, to take your place in the courtroom. Do you think you could do that for me?"

"Sure thing, John," I replied.

I was feeling nervous that things would not go as planned. How did I become the focus of this shot? I thought. The last thing I want now is to have this go wrong in front of Eric Peterson and Sonja Smits.

"Okay, let's do this. All take your places please," John called out.

There was a pause waiting for everyone to find their mark.

"Now on the count of 3, 2, 1, and … action!"

Carrie, played by Sonja Smits, began her walk down the main hall of the courthouse, followed by me. Just before she met Leon, played by Eric Peterson, I picked up speed and cut between them both, making my way into the courtroom.

"Cut. That was great, but let's do it one more time to make sure we have the shot. Everyone take your mark again."

I was feeling relieved that it all had worked out.

Just as I was making my way out of the courtroom and back to my mark, I found myself face to face with Sonja, who stopped and put her hand on her left hip.

"Girl, you really move in that chair. You have it all under control!"

I was shocked. She actually spoke to me!

Suddenly, I could hear John's voice once again.

"On the count of 3, 2, 1, and … action!"

I took to the floor once again, following Sonja in the same fashion as I had originally … down the courthouse hall, not long after I picked up speed, cutting between both her and Eric Peterson, before entering the courtroom.

"Cut. Great job everyone, we have that scene. Now let's move to scene twelve, episode three."

With the scene finished, I felt a sigh of relief. No longer needed on the set, I found a place off to the side and watched quietly as they continued to film.

At home later that evening I took a moment to reflect. I felt a real sense of accomplishment about my day. Not only had I gained the pleasure of working with two of Canada's most recognized television stars, I would be making a signature mark in the television series myself with a full-on view of the wheelchair. I knew this show aired nationally. I was now very grateful for the many positives in my life, happy to have found a new purpose. A purpose, it now seemed, I was having great success in achieving.

Chapter 14: My Ski Challenge in Kelowna

I finally found my efforts to promote the disabled community making their way through various mediums. With my modelling work now circulating through The Bay and Sears catalogues, and having landed a recurring role on Street Legal, I was becoming more of a public figure. I was approached through CADS (Canadian Association of Disabled Skiers) to do some promotional work. They were hoping to reach out to the disabled community to promote mono skiing.

Mono skiing is a way of hitting the slopes for individuals who use a wheelchair as their main mode of getting around. It uses a bucket-like seat that sits on a spring and is attached to a downhill ski. It allows those who have paralysis a daring chance to ski.

Thrilled with the opportunity, I agreed I would travel with a team to Kelowna, British Columbia and try to adapt to the sport while the cameras were rolling. I approached my mother first with the news. I knew my family would be initially apprehensive about my heading out west to ski. It was a sport I'd done poorly in even when I was on two feet.

"Mom, I've accepted an invitation to go skiing out in Kelowna, British Columbia," I stated, as I entered the dining room with hesitation, knowing my plans would be met with her uncertainty.

"You've what?" my mother responded.

"That's right. I've been invited to join the Canadian Association for Disabled Skiers in British Columbia. They'll be out there for a week of skiing and want me to join them to promote the sport of mono skiing."

"Mono skiing? What the heck is mono skiing? Don't tell me you're going to attempt to ski down a mountain, paralyzed from the waist down. Wendy, you know how your last attempt to ski down a hill ended. I think you should think carefully about accepting such a proposal, unless you have a death wish."

My mother was referring to my Grade Seven school trip to Honey Pot ski resort. It was on the mogul hill, an area we were warned to stay away from, where I took a devastating fall. I'd been trying to rescue a classmate who had fallen on the hill; the result left the two of us with broken legs and on crutches for the duration of the winter.

"Mom, I don't see it that way. I'll be joining a group of people, many of whom are wheelchair users, and I think the week would be exciting. It's an opportunity to meet some very interesting people while trying something new and challenging. I don't see the discouraging side to any of this."

At this point my sister joined us in the dining room, curious about the discussion.

"What's up? You'd think someone was getting ready for root canal. Why so serious?" she asked.

"It would appear your sister has decided to tempt her fate further," my mother explained. "There seems to be a part of her up for the challenge of mono skiing, hardly a safe sport, and she'll be hitting the mountain tops to pursue it."

"Do tell more! You've piqued my interest now," my sister added.

"I've been invited to Kelowna, British Columbia to do some publicity in the hope of attracting more wheelchair users to the sport of mono skiing."

"Is that the ski attached to the bucket, with arm braces used to steer it down the hill? I saw it on the internet. I was wondering about some of the activities you could still take part in while using your wheelchair. I think it's great you plan on trying it out. In fact, I just might join you, if that would be in any way possible. It's been a while since I've been skiing and I'd love to see Kelowna. What do ya say, sis?"

Kim worked at Canadian Airlines, so her flying pass would get her there free of charge.

"Great idea! I'll have to speak with the organizers but I see no reason why you couldn't join us. The room will be paid for, but you'll have to look after the fees at the slopes."

"That sounds like a fair plan to me. When do we leave?"

"There should be more information coming to me anytime. I'm really looking forward to it now. I think it's great that you're willing to join me. That will make the trip that much more enjoyable," I added.

"Let's hope you succeed on the hill this time around," my sister was quick to respond.

Packing was one chore I knew I had to take on, and I did so with hesitation. It did not help that many of my winter clothes were all packed away in the crawl space, so I enlisted my mother to lend a hand at gathering all that I would need: ski jacket, ski pants, and a number of turtleneck sweaters for a start. I knew I would have to keep warm somehow and the clothing I chose to bring along would be one way of assuring the temperatures did not get the best of me. Many sweaters, long john underwear, and flannel pajamas were all chosen as I prepared for the trip.

Early the following morning I received the final itinerary, giving me a better idea of what the days would entail. It explained more about the Canadian Association for Disabled Skiing, the organization hosting what they called the "Ski Challenge." It identified all the events that would take place throughout the week, although it was decided my services, mainly for publicly promoting the sport, would not be needed for the full week.

***

We flew to British Columbia on a direct flight out of Toronto's Pearson International Airport and landed in the evening. While we had flown into Kelowna, the Silver Star Ski Resort was located near Silver Star Provincial Park in the Shuswap Highlands of the Monashee Mountains. It was approximately twenty kilometres outside of the city of Vernon.

"Now this is a heavenly sight," I commented, as we drove through the maze-like roads. The scenery was breathtaking. The mountains surrounded the roads; it almost felt we were being swallowed by their height and the depths of the terrain surrounding us. It was early evening and the sun was setting on the hills, the scenery ablaze from the strength of the sun as it glared on the curves and ridges that formed the mountains around us.

"You bet it is, and we're not even on the mountain yet. It will only get better with an aerial view," my sister was quick to add.

"Let's just get there already, the anticipation is killing me. This is my first time out here in the Rockies and I'm excited to see all that it has to offer. Skiing aside, it would be nice to take in some of the atmosphere and culture outside of the resort while we're here, although I know our schedule is tight."

"That would be great, Wendy, although the resort sounds very accommodating, with workout rooms, a health spa, and a number of restaurants. I had a chance to go through the brochure and was impressed by all that it has to offer for the few days we are here."

The drive to Vernon was definitely a memorable experience. I continued to take in the sights as we drove along the highway. It was a time of reflection for me as to how far I had come on my journey. I had put my efforts forward in exposing the issue of disability. Efforts, it seemed, that were now truly paying off. I had done plenty of work publicly and I was now making a name for myself. Attracting the attention of CADS to have me promote the sport of mono skiing to the physically challenged community only reinforced the results of those efforts.

Arriving at the resort seemed a long-awaited reality and everyone there proved to be very receptive. Being a guest of the CADS organization put me front and centre; I would be one of the many representing the Ski Challenge publicly, and I learned how the four-day event would unfold. There would be press attending, and that is where I would come into play. I was there to experience the sport as a beginner, opening the activity to all wheelchair-bound individuals who were in search of a more active winter sport.

It was George Atkins, who was aware of my public efforts to expose the disability issue, who had commissioned me to be part of the event. It would be through his direction that the press would be governed. While I had met George briefly in Toronto, we had developed a kinship through emails and telephone calls, which we had made almost daily working up to the event. George was the first to greet both Kim and me upon our arrival at the Silver Star Ski Resort.

"Welcome Wendy," he said. "It's my pleasure to see you've finally arrived. I'm hoping you both had an enjoyable flight here."

"Oh yes, George, the flight was nice, but even more spectacular was the wonderful drive through Kelowna and into Vernon. I've never seen such mountains, a real scenic tour."

"Glad to hear you both had an opportunity to take in the sights, and yes Wendy, the scenery is breathtaking. Now it's time to get down to some real work, most of which will take place tomorrow when you head up the mountain. How are you feeling about that?" he asked.

"I'm looking forward to the challenge. As you know, I've yet to take on the sport of mono skiing and hope to succeed at it. I know my family will be relieved to see these next few days behind me. I had little success skiing prior to my accident, even on two legs," I explained.

"I'll have you know two of our best instructors will be looking after you while you're on the hill," George assured me. "I have personally chosen them, knowing their expertise will help you catch on to the technique for mono skiing. It takes guts to do what you have agreed to do, so getting the best people to instruct you was paramount. I'm positive you'll agree that they have this sport nailed."

"That's reassuring now that I'm here. There's no turning back now, George," I replied.

The next morning I met with my assigned instructors. "Well, good morning to you both," I began, trying to sound confident, although I was not quite ready for what was awaiting me. "I understand there'll be some instruction on this mono skiing sport, and no one better qualified to share the secrets than the two of you."

"That's right, Wendy, and no better time than now to introduce ourselves. I'm Bob, a veteran of mono skiing, and this is Steve. He'll be our Ski-Doo driver, and he's here to offer additional direction once we get you up the mountain. It will take some time to get up there, but we'll make it."

Steve jumped in to offer more information about the day I would be facing.

"Depending on your skills, I would think our trips up and down this mountain will be plenty. What level of injury are you, Wendy? Do you have any balance? It can really help with staying up on the ski."

I wasn't sure that I had exactly what it would take to keep me up on the odd looking piece of equipment.

"Yes, Steve, I do have pretty good balance, and I'm pleasantly surprised to hear that will give me an advantage riding down the mountain on this thing. I'm not sure of the actual technique but I have done some downhill skiing before I was in the wheelchair."

I did not dare tell him the last time I had skied had resulted in a broken leg. Not long after our brief introductions I was directed to look up to the mountain top, where there was a mono ski coming down the side of the mountain. It was a beautiful sight. The ski moved from one side of the mountain to the other, with the snow flying high behind the tail of the ski. It looked simply breathtaking. The motion was very smooth and precise and many people standing at the base of the hill took in the sight. The skier had what are called outriggers in both hands with little skis on them that are moved forward and away from the body to direct the mono ski. It was all very mesmerizing, better than a ballet performance.

"Now that's where we hope to take you this afternoon, up to the top of the mountain with nothing but blue skies and powdered snow for miles. Is it something you're interested in, Wendy?"

My nerves were growing more frazzled, but I did not let them get the best of me at that point.

"Gentlemen, let's take this just one step at a time. Getting me into the ski would be a great place to start."

Bob took hold of the mono ski, and prepared it so I could mount it. Gaining entrance into the bucket was hard on the hips, with both men lifting me, but a snug fit was necessary to ensure proper handling of the ski once in motion. I was tightly buckled into the ski and handed the outriggers to help me remain stable and in an upright position.

"Where to now, boys?" I quipped, confident in my ability to maintain firm grounding while sitting still in the ski. "If we're heading up that mountain for this afternoon I suggest we get a move on."

Bob and Steve looked impressed with my initial stability and Bob skied behind me, pushing me and the mono ski toward the Ski-Doo. Steve was on the machine and waiting to pull us both up the mountain.

"I'll be back here to anchor you," Bob explained, crouching down behind the mono ski, both hands on either side of the bucket. And on that note, the Ski-Doo began to rev and I was handed a rope to grasp while we slowly headed toward the hill.

My excitement was mixed with a great deal of hesitation and trepidation. On one hand I looked forward to the new experience, climbing the mountain and seeing the many sights on the long way up. On the other hand I had not had the best experience in my last attempt at skiing. Would this trip up the mountain be disastrous, with my only memory to take home being my failure to accomplish the full route down the mountain? God forbid I break any bones. I decided we'd have to leave it up to fate and good intentions, as we slowly worked our way up the hill, Bob holding on to the bucket and me with my outriggers at both sides of the mono ski balancing me as the Ski-Doo pulled us both forward.

A quarter of the way up Steve stopped the Ski-Doo and Bob made sure I was stable before letting go of both sides of the bucket. I appeared to be sitting tall independently with my overall balance much less impaired, thanks to the return of sensation in my lower extremities.

"Why have we stopped?" I asked. We had clearly more than three-quarters of the hill left to climb.

"Well Wendy, we figure we'll start you out at a level that won't prove too complicated seeing as you've never been on a mono ski before," Bob explained

"Yeah Wendy, let's take this one step at a time here," Steve added.

At that point Bob took the back of the bucket and turned me around so I was facing down the hill.

"There's no time like the present to test out your balance. Are you ready to take on the hill?" he asked.

I saw no way but down at that point.

"Yes, let's go for it!"

Bob pushed forward on the mono ski and down the hill I started, Bob holding a rope attached to the bucket. With no time to think I put both outriggers down in the snow to support me, although my fear rose as the speed of the ski increased and my control of it diminished.

"Yiiiikes, help me Bob, I'm picking up too much speed!" I yelled, as I accelerated down the hill, my hair blowing in the wind and my eyes swelling with tears from the speed.

Suddenly Bob pulled on the tether, slowing me down so I could get a better handle on the ride. It was scary, but also an exhilarating challenge. The outriggers were definitely a great help in keeping me upright, and the bucket was equipped with a shock absorbent spring, offering a smoother ride over the bumps that I skied across.

"You're doing great, Wendy," Bob yelled. "The outriggers are there for support and I can see you're getting the hang of it. Keep it up and we'll make it to the top of the hill before the end of the day!"

My balance was spot on. The only problem was the speed that came with each recovery from a near fall. Each time I straightened up my steering going downhill, the mono ski began to go faster. The only way to stop now was to fall, and how could I do that without hurting myself or breaking any bones?

"Do something Bob, I'm losing control here!" I yelled back at him. "I have no idea how to stop this thing."

Not long after my distress call I felt a tighter pull on the tether attached to the ski, slowing down my speed and better preparing me for a complete stop. Bob was definitely an expert skier and needed little effort to control us both. He immediately began working on stopping the two of us.

"Wow! This thing really moves," was my first response after coming to a complete stop. "I've never experienced anything like it. I've been on a number of rides in my time that have yet to offer the thrill that one just did."

"I have to say I'm impressed with your control of the ski, Wendy. It'll be no time before you're doing these hills with precise strokes of the outriggers, offering you a more streamlined process. Your balance is spot on," Bob said.

"We've brought up quite a few newcomers to this sport, and on this hill," added Steve. "I have to say, your balance is quite impressive. Working on the technique of leaning side to side on the ski while using the outriggers as support is how you'll master it. You're proving to be a quick learner."

"I'm very pleased to hear that, gentlemen. When do you think we'll be ready to try out some real hills?" I questioned.

Both Bob and Steve looked at each other, before Bob replied to my statement.

"Now Wendy, we want you to make it off this hill today in one piece. Let's take it one step at a time, or should I say one mountain at a time. We have a few days ahead of us, plenty of time to get you groomed and further up the mountain."

Bob was right. But there was something more important suddenly. With all of the excitement I had experienced, my bladder was in need of a washroom.

"Let's get you pointed in the right direction here, Wendy, and make it down to the club house. You've definitely proven you have what it takes on these hills. Maybe after some lunch we'll come back up here, and head a little further up the hill," Steve said.

We made our way down the mountain with ease. There were many skiers passing us on their way down to the bottom of the hill. The scenery was beautiful, as I had suspected it would be, with our surroundings covered in fresh white snow, with not a square inch of green land showing for miles.

The Canadian Association for Disabled Skiers - National Capital Division, known as CADS-NCD, was founded in October 1979. It is dedicated to assisting individuals with a disability to lead active lives through participation in skiing and snowboarding. CADS has divisions across Canada and usually come together through events like the annual Ski Challenge, held at various venues within the boundaries of Canada, like Silver Star Ski Resort. Members competing in the annual Ski Challenge event that week all lived with various forms of physical challenges that included paralysis and amputations as well as those with visual impairments.

Back at the clubhouse, I was reunited with my sister and ready for some lunch. I found the fresh air to be draining and it helped work up an appetite. There were endless choices and my decision making was not at its best.

"Are you hungry for something substantial?" my sister asked as we both took a seat at a vacant booth and browsed the menu.

"Are you kidding? I could eat a horse right now. I'm famished."

Music playing in the background began to get louder, and the atmosphere became almost jovial. Hands began to clap and many started cheering out loud. Not long after the cheering became almost unbearable, a group of young men made their way to the dance floor, all putting down a pitcher of beer prior to their journey through the crowds. It was then that the clapping took on a beat-like tempo, and they all started chanting "1, 2, 3, 4." I looked over my shoulder to see one of the young men jumping on his right leg, with his left leg, it seemed, sliding down his pant leg.

Then his prosthetic leg came sliding out of his pants!

The cheering became louder and the crowd began to laugh out loud.

The focus then turned to two more of the young men, dancing to the beat of the chants. This time it was both their left arms that they began waving in the air, high above their heads. They waved them back and forth from left to right until suddenly they both lost their prosthetic arms onto the dance floor.

This was like something out of the movies! The crowds were now outrageously excited and reactive. It was not long before someone made their way quickly to the dance floor with a wheelchair to rescue the one-legged bandit from falling flat on his face. Not long after that, the dance floor appeared to fill up with others who were interested in joining in on the fun. Many of them were now grooving to the beat of the music, and there were continued chants with many holding hands and circling around the amputees that had put on the show. The feel of the room was fluid as those now on the dance floor began waving their arms in the air while dancing to the beat. The chanting subsided, but not the crowd. All those who made their way onto the dance floor continued to keep to the beat with nothing holding them back in the dance moves category. It was really quite a sight!

"What are we witnessing here?" I blurted out, after observing such a raw display of acceptance throughout the room. It was like nothing I had seen before and definitely forced me to delve deeper into thought.

George Atkins had made it clear before I agreed to join the CADS group out west, that they were an exceptional group of people. Many had come through much of what I had, whether it was a motor vehicle accident, diving mishap, or some other unforeseen tragedy. Others would have eyesight impairments. He certainly was not exaggerating when he said I would be impressed by the group and feel like I could fit in. A group of individuals with no pretense about their disability, and certainly feeling no limitations as far as what they could do despite their physical challenges.

I had decided what they displayed was their ability to have fun with their circumstances, almost to exploit it. They were in a place where everyone could relate to each other on some level and let it all happen in a way most of us could find humour in, not insult. All too often people are intimidated by the limitations of others and therefore situations can very likely become almost awkward. With everyone in the room, aside from resort staff, CAD administration, and guests brought to the Ski Challenge, we could all genuinely laugh and have fun with the physical side of what made the trip to Silver Star Ski Resort possible. And that was our disabilities.

Not long after the exhibition was over I noticed George searching through the crowd to find me, wondering what my reaction to what we had just witnessed might be. I quickly waved over to him, and winked, to let him know I had approved, in fact enjoyed what some may have found a little too much as far as having fun with the topic of disability. But who better to display such an enlightening side of living with a disability than those doing just that?

George made his way over.

"Well Wendy, was I wrong when I said this was a very dynamic crowd you'd be meeting here on the West Coast?"

"I should say not," I quickly replied. "I found it all quite moving, a little daring, but definitely humorous. Is this an annual routine or something that came out of the blue?"

"Well, there are few traditions that could top that," George responded, with a look of guilt on his face. He might have warned me of the exhibition that was coming, given it was a tradition, and a tradition many would find quite shocking.

My sister Kim joined in the conversation.

"I thought it was fabulous, and who better to have fun with the subject than the people living it, day in, day out."

"I know, you're right," I said. "Now that we've got that out of the way, George are there any other situations that might come up that we should be forewarned about? This is definitely a lively crowd. I wouldn't want to see myself losing faith in them, or you."

"No ladies, there are no more real shockers to come. Besides that, I've yet to hear how your morning on the hill went today. Really Wendy, how did you find it all? With all of this excitement, I never thought to question you about it."

I was quick to respond.

"There were so many moments I thought I'd kill you for getting me involved in all of it, but then going down that mountain like a bolt of lightning gave me a feeling of daring excitement that I have never experienced before. I've mastered my balance on the ski, so it now comes down to refining the actual technique. I'm told that is the biggest challenge. Any tips George?"

"I am busting with admiration at all the participants here at the challenge this week. The mono skiers and visually impaired in particular," George said. "That doesn't mean I would try it myself, or have any insights to pass on to you, Wendy. But as I made clear to you earlier, you have the best instructors up here at your disposal. You can trust in the direction they offer and I'm confident you will only get better with time."

We were quick to finish our meals amidst the excitement of the room. People were coming and going now, with the ski hills a priority. It had been a full year since the last CADS communal and many were craving the exhilaration of flying down the slopes.

With my own morning on the hill counted a success, we decided the afternoon would be dedicated to the press, both print and television. The majority of them were local; the CTV camera crew travelling with us was the only out of town coverage. The interviews seemed endless, although I was happy to offer my insights: mono skiing was a viable sport for those daring enough to face the challenge. I knew that getting word out on this could inspire many individuals. After finishing with the media, Kim and I made our way back to our room.

"Well, that was certainly a day," my sister stated, exhausted.

"You can say that again! I've never seen hills so mammoth. Mono skiing was a difficult task to take on. I'm quite proud of myself."

"And you should be. I am very proud of you, not just on your mono skiing but on how you've pulled your life together. Look how it all began and where you are today. As a family, your accident paralyzed us all. We were so worried for you.

"Oh gosh, Wendy," she went on, "you were so active before the accident. Your dancing was part of who you were. It should have been any one of us but you, we thought at first. We were petrified over how things would work out for you. And look at you now!"

"That's very kind of you, Kim, and I am glad you shared it. I rarely look back on things. I guess I'm trying my best to continually move forward."

"And you've done it all so gracefully. I know there have been times of frustration and anger but you've always found a way to overcome any sense of helplessness, and you've triumphed as a result. You have a lot to be proud of, my dear sister."

"It's funny you should say that. My relationship with God has had some questionable moments throughout this whole ordeal. But at times, when things are good like now, I almost feel like all this was meant to be, part of a plan."

Kim looked puzzled.

"Designed to put me here to help make a difference for people in wheelchairs," I finished.

"I guess that's one way of looking at it," Kim responded.

It was the first time I had shared this belief with anyone, although it was a thought I had often. Many young women would kill to be doing what I, just by chance, had fallen into. The modelling jobs were relatively steady now and my work on Street Legal continued at intervals. I had a lot to be grateful for.

The next three days continued to impress me. The skiers I watched coming down the mountainside literally took my breath away. They manoeuvred themselves so gracefully and definitively that anyone watching was sure to admire their skill. As for me, it was not until my last day on the slopes I was able to make it down without a tumble. While I was not so quick to pick up on the mono skiing technique, the whole experience moved me and remains in my mind along with vivid recollections of all that I witnessed throughout my stay at Silver Star Mountain Resort.

Chapter 15: Landing a Job at YTV

One day I was preparing to go out with some friends when the telephone rang.

"Well look at that, I caught you at home," said a voice I didn't recognize.

"I'm sorry?"

"It's me, you fool. Sia! It's been a long time."

"Oh my God, I can't believe it. How the heck are you doing?" I asked.

Sia was a friend who had often visited me while I was in the Toronto Western Hospital. She was a full-time student at Ryerson University and was taking a radio and television course. She hoped to become a producer. I was a little taken aback; it had been years since we had last spoken.

"I am doing fine," Sia replied, "and by the looks of things, you are too. I see you everywhere these days."

"Well I can't take that away from you. My agent, Rhona, is hard at work trying to find me jobs and her efforts are finally beginning to pay off. What about you Sia, what keeps you busy these days?"

"I'm now at YTV. I finally landed that producer's job you know I've wanted since my days at Ryerson. It all fell into place for me. I have been here for three years now."

"That's great news, Sia. I'm so happy that things have worked out for you."

"Yes, things couldn't be better right now. I was wondering if you'd be available to get together anytime soon. It's been so long and you have definitely a lot of news to share with me."

I had some time free so we decided to meet the next day at a coffee shop close to the YTV studios. It had probably been four years since we had talked. I had returned to school and Sia was busy trying to get her career off the ground.

Before heading to the coffee shop I called to make sure access would not be a problem and that parking was available. It was easy getting there; the real challenge came with finding a parking space that would accommodate my wheelchair. I circled the block a number of times before locating a good spot. But it involved parallel parking.

This is not an easy task when driving with hand controls. My right hand has to control the gas and my left hand is fully occupied with the steering wheel. Having the mirrors positioned properly is a must to ensure I don't hit the other parked cars. I remember parking parallel that day because it was my only option. It took a few tries but I finally succeeded in manoeuvering the car into its place. Sia was already inside the coffee shop when I arrived at the front door.

"Hello my friend, it's great to see you!" Sia looked really good. She had put on a little weight that definitely agreed with her, and her hair was longer than I remembered. She had a rugged way about her that was made more obvious when she greeted me with a firm handshake.

"It's been too long, Wendy. What a pleasure it is to see you looking so well."

"The pleasure came with your telephone call, Sia. It's been too long."

"Now tell me all that you've been up to, Wendy. How on earth did you find yourself in the world of modelling? Kudos to you, girlfriend!"

"Instead of returning to my job at Domtar, I decided to go back to school. I enrolled in a business admin course at Sheridan College, which offered me the flexibility to do other things.

"Business administration, how'd you like the course?"

"The course was great. But I have to say, Sia, I was faced with some challenges socially at times after I left hospital. I felt the disabled community needed a platform, a place for inclusion. Not long afterward, I found an agent. She's been great to work with and we've been fortunate with the public response."

"That's fabulous to hear, Wendy. I know change doesn't always come easy. Glad to see you are making your mark. How's the family?"

"Everyone is doing great. You know we moved into a new home all adapted for the wheelchair. There's an elevator that brings me to all levels of the home, with ramps around back. I couldn't ask for more. They've all been great through the transition. There were some rough times for me. Regaining my independence took some work but I feel I am there now."

"Was it really difficult, Wendy?"

"I faced some really dark days in the beginning. The loss of Grania is a reality that has never left me. I feel her spirit in all that I do. She is with me every day. Now about you...." I quickly added to pick up the mood. "Tell me more about your job with YTV."

"Well, I joined them shortly after finishing my course at Ryerson. There's a really great group of people here and I'm enjoying the pace. Which brings me to the reason for my call. How busy are you nowadays?"

"That would depend on the day. Why, what are you thinking?"

"We've just launched a new show. It's called Street Noise, aimed at teens thirteen to eighteen, topics across the board. I'd really love to see you on the show somehow, Wendy."

"You're kidding! But Sia, I have so little background in the television industry. I'd be like a wet noodle."

"That's why we have what are called field producers, Wendy, who make sure our on-air talent get it all right while out in the field. I really do think you're the perfect fit for this, and the wheelchair only adds to your selling features for the show. The kids see you have a disability, but you're not letting it stop you."

"Why, that's the whole reason I've been modelling Sia, to expose the issue. You might be right here. I would love to be part of this production!"

I could not believe this was happening.

"I wanted to talk to you before I ran it past the executive producer of the show, Stephanie Wright, but I know she'll love the concept. It just makes so much sense."

"Well I am definitely on board, Sia. I think it's an awesome opportunity."

We sat together for more than an hour over coffee, and it was like no time had passed. Sia was very perceptive about life, as she'd showed when she thought of me for the show. She was gifted with a very warm and caring heart and was out to make a difference in the world. She felt she could do that through television.

I received a telephone call from her not long after our meeting, confirming I would be a part-time field reporter for Street Noise on YTV.

My career was on a real upswing, with modelling now taking up much of my time. Jobs for The Bay, Eaton's, and Sears catalogue were coming regularly now, along with part-time work with YTV as a segment reporter. There was little time to dwell on the small stuff, and my mission of promoting the issue of wheelchairs and the disabled community seemed to take on a life of its own.

Chapter 16: The Pageant

Venus Swimwear is a reputable American company that sponsors pageants in the United States. It took some work, but organizers were able to bring the events to venues in Canada. The pageants are held across the country, with finalists brought together for the international finals, which were to be held in Boca Raton, Florida that year. The Toronto pageant was scheduled to take place at the Sutton Place Hotel, and I was entered. I planned to meet Rhona there prior to the competition to go over my recent jobs and collect payment for work completed. I had been hesitant to enter the pageant but Rhona had assured me it would be a great career move.

I dressed for the occasion, sporting a crisp white shirt with a black cigarette pant. While the outfit was classic, I wore a black bolero hat to add a bit of style to the ensemble. The wheelchair often garnered attention, but the hat really set my look off. I looked like I had wheeled right off the fashion runway of Milan.

Not long after entering the auditorium, I was greeted by Rhona.

"Well, what have we here? You've come all decked out, and you look fabulous!" was her initial reaction.

"Just thought I'd do something a little different for this evening," I replied.

After finding seats at a table we both ordered glasses of chilled chardonnay and began catching up with all the work I had done that week. There had been two Bay shoots and the reporting gig for YTV.

"I've had a busy week, Rhona, with tonight bringing an end to it all."

"How did the photo shoots for The Bay go?" Rhona asked. "I assume you worked with Mary Jo?"

"I was there Tuesday and Thursday of this week with a tentative shoot coming up in the next two weeks. She said she'd be in touch with you. The real challenge came with trying to squeeze in a story for YTV. The topic was overcoming adversity, and there were four young girls who took part. Their stories were really moving."

"Were you able to complete the segment?" Rhona asked.

"Yes, the story is in the can and ready to air."

At that point we were joined by the organizer of the pageant, Judy Rusnell, who came over to our table with instructions for me about how the evening would unfold.

"Good evening, ladies, I see you're indulging in a glass of courage before things begin. Most participants have arrived and are in the dressing room preparing. Wendy, I do hope you're still planning to compete this evening."

"Yes, it's my intention to, although pageants aren't something I know much about. This is all new to me. I'm not quite sure what the evening will entail, other than at some point tonight I'll be sporting a two-piece swimsuit," I replied.

Judy explained that there would be twelve women competing, with three rounds of competition: women's active wear, swimwear, and finally an evening gown segment. She reminded us that the swimsuits would be supplied but all competitors were responsible for supplying their own outfits for the other two segments.

Judy insisted we get moving and began leading the way to the dressing room designated for the contestants. After following her down a long corridor I was escorted into the change room, where eleven girls were already busy prepping themselves for the competition.

"Okay ladies, we're down to the final hours," Judy announced, as I began unpacking my things.

It was awkward as I entered the change room. The reactions of the other girls to seeing me in a wheelchair were mixed, although I had desensitized myself to such stares during my modelling work. Not everyone was prepared to accept the wheelchair, considering the glamour often associated with modelling; I had found that some of the people I worked with still pursued absolute perfection. I wondered if tonight would be any different.

I began laying out my outfits and preparing my makeup and hair care products when I was approached by one of the other girls.

"Hello and welcome," she said, sounding optimistic and friendly. "I'm Kate."

"Hello, Kate," I responded, happy to know not everyone was out to kill. "I'm Wendy. Is this your first pageant?" I added, to keep the conversation going.

"Yes, and it might well be my very last, given the nerves that have come on the last hour and a half. I believe I've done my hair six times over, and I haven't found one style I like. It looks like this could be a long night."

"Your hair looks fine," I answered. "Relax, it's only hair! This is my first pageant too."

Kate appeared to be in her early twenties with brown hair, close to shoulder length. She wore it in a short bob cut, and it had a natural wave to it. She was quite tall at about five foot ten. She wore a pair of Calvin Klein jeans and a T-shirt, which gave her a more casual appearance than many of us there. I recall how nice it was to be approached by Kate, offering a more cordial feel to the evening. There were ten other girls in the change room; however, we had little chance to mingle, and everyone appeared nervous. We were all there for the moment, and the competition. Later on, I was impressed by the kindness we all shared toward each other as we went through the evening.

The evening began with the active wear segment of the competition.

I had put together a tennis outfit that would show a realistic activity for someone in a wheelchair to participate in. Many people in wheelchairs play tennis. In fact, it's one of the few sports that need little, if any, adjustment in order to play the game. It can be played directly from the wheelchair, with the net height and swing the important factors. I'd had the opportunity to play a few times. The sport's realistic attributes were what drew me to it as a sport to try, not to mention the cute little outfits available to play in. An outfit and tennis racquet were all I needed to complete the segment. My hair was up in a ponytail, with a white skirt and polo T-shirt to complete the sporty look.

Although getting to the stage proved a bit nerve wracking, a ramp was set up along the right side of the stage offering me access, and it was at an appropriate incline that I could climb the ramp independently. The music was loud and my heart pounded, almost in tune to the drums echoing throughout the room. The fear brought on exhilaration as I found myself onstage with what seemed a million eyes glaring at me while I did my best to keep to the beat of the music. I posed with the tennis racquet at my shoulder, swung it out in front of me, before placing it on my lap and moving around the stage to ensure no one in the audience missed getting a full-on view of my sporty attire. I entered the stage seventh of the twelve girls competing. I never looked back once and faced the audience with a smile worn ear to ear in an attempt to hide the intense fear I was feeling.

There were five judges sitting in front of the stage, their eyes planted on me. I remember making eye contact with a middle-aged woman in the centre row of the audience. She became a place to focus my attention, my look, my smile. She had a comforting appearance that I gravitated to and she remained my focal point throughout the competition.

The swimwear segment was easy since the competition was sponsored by Venus Swimwear, with colour and style up to the contestant. I had chosen a two-piece design, with bold colours prominent in both the top and bottom of the swimsuit. Making my way up the ramp to the stage I again felt my heart pound, almost in sync to the music, with an exhilaration hard to describe. The blood flow throughout my body was intense, with the music and audience only adding to the excitement. I could hardly breathe, and the feeling was even stronger as I made circles around the stage while displaying the bikini chosen to be worn that segment. I stayed focused on the woman in the audience to keep my centre place on stage and pushed myself forward with long strokes again, while keeping in time with the beat of the music. I added a few wheelchair wheelies to give my presentation a little pep and received a great response from the crowd with applause and whistles streaming through the auditorium.

The final segment was formal wear. I had decided on a simple black dress but wore the bolero hat with it. This gave me a different appeal from the other contestants and it dressed up my final look. I wore my hair down straight and behind my ears, giving more focus to the dress and hat. My jewellery was simple: gold studs for earrings and a chain-link bracelet on my right wrist. I wore a simple pair of black pumps to finish the outfit.

With the first two segments out of the way, the mood was much less tense, and the music playing in the background calmed the atmosphere. The competition now appeared to become more sophisticated, with many of the girls showing a refined style while appearing more at ease on stage; there was less tension, and many of us were now finding it fun to focus on the elegance we displayed with our choice of gowns. The first two rounds had been the stepping stone to the grand finale.

Following the final round, Kate and I were able to connect and discuss what we had experienced onstage and whether the judges were impressed with what they saw.

"Well, how do you think you did?" was my first question to Kate while we were putting away our outfits.

"It's not how well I did, I'm just glad it's over," Kate replied. "I don't recall ever feeling so much excitement, and I'm not sure it's something I'd want to experience again."

"Really Kate, it was that overwhelming?" I asked.

"My breathing was shallow, more than I care to remember and the music was hard to keep up to at times. I felt like I was running on empty at times – more obviously in the first two rounds of competition. I was uncomfortable while I was trying to pretend there was no other place I'd rather be. I don't believe I'm a natural at any of this pageantry business, although my agent believes the more I expose myself to these elements, the more likely they will become second nature. And you, Wendy, how did you find the experience? How do you think you did?"

There was so much going on in my head it was hard to put any of it into words right away. I had competed in a swimsuit pageant, perhaps helping the judges and audience see beyond merely how I get around in my wheelchair. The overall experience was moving and one that I would not take back. This was all in my attempt to make a difference in the limiting attitudes I often faced. I was glad it was over and that I was able to meet the challenge. I had to be honest in my response to Kate.

"I found it to be a thrilling experience," I answered. "Something I've never felt before but it was more for a reason."

"Really, Wendy?"

"My wheelchair is often challenged by social attitudes and it's been my hope to show the abilities we have rather than the limitations that are often placed on us. Unfortunately, it's society that often limits us, not necessarily ourselves."

"Why, you're right. I never thought about it that way."

"Knowing there is no way out of the wheelchair for me makes it more logical to try my best to make it work for me. That means taking on challenges like this and seeing where they take me. I cannot change what is, I can only learn to adapt and perhaps challenge myself. What's that Nike phrase? *Just do it!*"

"You've definitely got the right attitude, Wendy. I am sure you shocked a lot of people out there doing what you did. Competing in this pageant took guts!" Kate responded.

The real test in patience was waiting for the judges to make their final decision. We all gathered in a large room, much like a banquet hall. The twelve very nervous participants all waited to hear who would go on to represent Canada in the international competition.

There were some awkward moments as we waited. Some contestants, I was sure, were wondering why I had even bothered entering the competition. It wasn't so much what they said, but the way they acted. Many of them had no idea I was an actual model with many print ads to my credit, but the judges knew this through my biography and portfolio. I also had my part-time job at YTV that put me in the spotlight. I was actually one of the more professionally established contestants in the competition, with a real shot at winning as far as Rhona was concerned.

After waiting a short time for the judges to finalize their decisions, we were all called out to the stage in the order we competed. I resumed my seventh position and we sat on the stage, with the judges seated directly in front of us. The master of ceremonies took the envelope that revealed the runners-up and the ultimate winner. We would all collectively hold hands while the MC prepared to reveal those girls who had placed in the event.

He began with the third runner-up.

"Ladies, it is with great pleasure that I prepare to reveal those lucky ladies that have placed in this competition. I can assure you the judges had their hands full when trying to narrow this down to just four of you. It was no easy task. Without further ado, I'd like to call Whitney Krantz to the stage, and congratulations on your third runner-up position."

The audience and the contestants all began to clap while Whitney made her way up to the stage. She did appear to be nervous, but very excited about placing. They handed her flowers and she took her place on the stage.

"Now it's time for the second runner-up. I assure you all, this choice was no easier than the third runner-up."

It was comical how he prolonged the inevitable announcement of her name, keeping everyone on their guard while waiting to hear who he would call.

"Would Vanessa David please make her way up to the stage? Congratulations Vanessa, you have taken the position of second runner-up this evening."

The screams could not be missed! Vanessa David went into hysterics after hearing her name called and the rest of the guests were aghast at the pitch of her screams.

It was at that point that the MC announced the first and final runner-up to the title of Miss Venus International.

"Ladies and gentlemen, please put your hands together as I call tonight's first runner-up to the stage. Lisa Beattie, please come and take your place on the stage with the rest of these lucky ladies."

Lisa was much more subdued than the first two. She almost appeared too shocked to make it to her position on stage.

With first, second, and third runners-up now introduced, the anticipation grew throughout the auditorium. "Now, ladies and gentlemen, is the moment we've all been anticipating. It is with the greatest of pleasures that I introduce you all to tonight's winner," he announced, while shuffling the envelope from one hand to the other, keeping everyone in suspense.

"It is with great pleasure that I announce to you all this year's winner of the 1993 Miss Venus Toronto is Miss Wendy Murphy. Wendy please, make your way here to the front of the stage." There was no way this could be happening! All of those difficult moments of competition suddenly came flashing back as I realized I was the winner. It would be me, Wendy Murphy, who would represent Canada in the international competition. I would be going to Boca Raton as a contestant, the first and only woman in a wheelchair to ever accomplish such a feat.

"That's right, folks," the MC was saying, "Wendy Murphy will take the title, and that's not all. Wendy, there's a full set of luxury luggage that will be awarded to you, a workout system by Medi-Flex, and there's also a fine Ricoh camera that is now yours. But more importantly, you'll receive an all-expense-paid trip to Boca Raton, Florida where you'll face off for the title of Miss Venus International."

Suddenly, I couldn't wait to share the news with my family! Rhona was right – the world was ready to see wheelchairs in a whole new light!

After packing up my things I went back to meet Rhona. I was surrounded by well-wishers and excited to contact my family. Judy Rusnell, the organizer, approached me first with words of encouragement.

"I'm so glad you didn't let your nerves hold you back, and my gut feeling was right. You're very accomplished and this win only proves that."

"I also was confident you had a great chance at taking home the title, Wendy," Rhona added.

"Thank you all for your encouragement, but right now I'd like to get in touch with my family to tell them the news. I know my father will be here any time now to pick me up but I want to call my mother to share my victory. I still can't believe it!"

At that moment I was passed a cellular telephone and proceeded to dial my family home. When my mother answered, I shared the good news.

"Mom, you're not going to believe it, but I've won. I won the pageant." My words were mixed with tears of joy while my mother congratulated me on my victory.

"Your father will be there shortly, Wendy. When you get home we'll celebrate your great achievement as a family!"

There was so much to be grateful for; not only had I taken first place but I would be going to Boca Raton as a contestant in the international competition! Is this all for real? I kept thinking. Could this actually be happening to me?

Not long after the phone call home to my mother, my father entered the room and with everyone surrounding me it didn't take him long to figure out what was happening.

I went on to explain to him that I had taken the title of Miss Venus Swimwear Toronto, that I would be moving on to the international competition. "It all sounds so exciting, Wendy," he replied. "I know you'll take it all in stride, as you have since taking on the jobs you have gotten through Rhona. I had a very good feeling that something would come of your efforts this evening. I know you've done a lot publicly and all for a great reason."

I knew that my father was talking about my mission. The modelling remained an important part of exposing the issue of inclusion, a way of telling the world that we are people first, who happened to have a disability. I was not only exposing the issue through print ads, but through television as well with my work on YTV. I wondered how my achievement this evening might help advance my mission.

The conversation continued as I transferred into the front seat of the car and my father folded up the wheelchair and placed it into the trunk.

"Well Wendy, you must feel proud of your accomplishment. I know we are all thrilled," he said, holding on to my hand in a tight grip, reassuring me of the family's support.

I felt a flurry of emotions as we made our way back home. I had never expected to place in the competition, let alone take the crown. I wanted people to see Wendy first, not the wheelchair, and it seemed that was exactly what had occurred. I believe I impressed many of the judges with my courage to be in the pageant at all, and it ended up paying off with a win. I was out to make a statement about just what individuals with a disability are capable of, and I had pulled it off successfully. Just how things would go in Florida, however, had me questioning my win.

"Dad, I'm feeling many emotions right now and it might take me a little time to process all of this. I'm not sure I'm ready to face an international competition."

"Wendy, when have you ever let fear stop you from what you hoped to accomplish? In fact, it's the perception many have that has put you on such a remarkable journey. It's been your hope to change those attitudes you're now facing. I say take this win for all that it's worth and let it work for you. The ball is in your court now, and I say you should roll with it, no pun intended."

He has a point, I thought. I had entered the competition to make a statement and not to win. As fate would have it, I had taken the crown, and it was now up to me to share my message internationally. Whether others were ready or not to see it, the message was now mine to share.

Before long we were home and I was greeted at the front door by my mom and brother, Jeff.

"Congratulations Wendy!" they yelled in sync with one another as I entered the front foyer from the elevator.

"Thank you, all of you, for your continued support," I responded. "There's so much to share, I hardly know where to start. In fact, maybe we'll leave it for tomorrow. I will have to work at YTV, unless the schedule has changed. I will know early in the morning. I'm supposed to call Sia and Phyllis by eight tomorrow morning and I'll have time after that to tell you about this evening. I am terribly tired and will be in better shape to share the details after a good night's sleep."

I went to bed with a lot to think about. It was incredibly overwhelming. I had entered the competition to make a difference and to help others get past the limitations often placed on us, not necessarily to win. I would now be taking on a much more significant responsibility, an international competition, and I had doubts about moving forward with it. Am I prepared to do this? I wondered. Would I go that step further and take on the international competition as I had the local? The competition would take me to Boca Raton the following week and I decided sleeping on it was the best thing I could do.

I woke early the following morning knowing I had to get in touch with my producers at YTV to find out my schedule. I called Sia, the producer of Street Noise, the show I did segments for. Sia came to the phone quickly when she heard it was me calling. Her voice was full of excitement.

"Wendy, I'm so glad you've called, I've got some pretty exciting news for you."

"Well, Sia," I responded, "I have some pretty incredible news too. I'll go first. Do you recall that pageant I decided to try my hand at? Well it took place last night. And I've taken the title, Sia. They crowned me Miss Venus Swimwear Toronto last night. I'm still a little numb from it all. I never, in my wildest dreams imagined myself as the winner."

"Wendy, that's great news!" Sia burst out. "What happens next? Is there another competition?"

"It now takes on an international flair. The competition will take place in Boca Raton, Florida at the end of next week, so I may need time away from the station. Now what's your news?"

"Wendy, Gloria Estefan has recovered from her bus accident and will be going on tour. *Into the Light* is her new album, all a reflection of her recovery and we'd like you to do the interview. She was fortunate the damage to her spinal cord was not permanent. She'll perform in Toronto next weekend and we're hoping to send you to collect the interview."

My mind began to race and I could not hold back my delight knowing I was the reporter they wanted for the interview. Not only had I won the pageant, I was now first in line to interview Gloria Estefan. The producers obviously felt I would be a great example for a young audience. While my spinal cord damage was permanent, I was certainly moving on with my life, and succeeding.

"That is a phenomenal suggestion," I replied. "I would be thrilled to interview Gloria Estefan about her recovery. I've read about it a number of times and know she's grateful to have fully recovered from her initial paralysis. How can we make this work, Sia? I would give up the pageant if I had to."

"Let's not get ahead of ourselves, Wendy. I will talk with Phyllis and see what can be done to make this work."

"You know I'll be flexible. I hope to see this happen, Sia. You have my full cooperation," I assured her.

Hanging up the telephone, I found myself in a state of disbelief about all that was happening in my life. My modelling work was circulating widely through flyers and catalogues for a number of Canadian department stores. I was now the winner of a pageant that I had little interest in pursuing professionally. And finally, my work through YTV could possibly have me sitting face to face with the international music star, Gloria Estefan, who proved the odds were on her side following a serious bus accident resulting in a broken back, although with no permanent paralysis. My life was definitely looking up. It seemed only a few years earlier I was clinging to the hope that my life would turn around, that I would find meaning and purpose to carry on. I was in the depths of loss; no Grania and paralyzed from the waist down. Through will and perseverance I had been able to overcome it all.

***

My week at the Venus International Competition in Boca Raton, Florida opened my eyes to the world of competitive pageants. It was culture shock for me to learn that these pageants were a career choice for many girls and women in the United States. For many who know the circuit there is money to be made, with modelling contracts, gifts, prizes, and cash just a few of the perks.

The woman who shared a room with me for the week had driven to four different states just to qualify for the competition. For those hoping for international recognition, cosmetic enhancements are common; breast implants are among the more prevalent procedures.

The week had us all busy interacting with each other. Our days began early, and competition behind the scenes was a constant presence. We were kept busy meeting with any one of the eight judges on the selection panel, sometimes in groups, sometimes individually. Our résumés and modelling portfolios were submitted for review; we were having classes on hair and makeup application; some remained busy practising their runway strut. Everyone was responsible for making it to production rehearsal. The producers choreographed a song and dance routine for all the girls to participate in, myself included, with wheelchair spins and wheelies. The week was a thrilling process that brought fifty-two beautiful young women together from around the world to show their talents and competitive sides.

While I did not take home the crown for the international competition, I was awarded the Contestants' Choice Award by the other competitors. We were all given the opportunity to vote for the young woman that we, as contestants, felt to be the most deserving of the title.

I had the pleasure of meeting many incredible women during the week of competition, and to receive such an honour from my peers meant more to me than any crown could have offered. I was truly moved. Once again I believed I had shown the world that life in a wheelchair did not restrict anyone from pursuing their dreams.

***

Because I was in Florida while Gloria Estefan was performing in Toronto, we decided that I would travel to Montreal to tape my interview with her.

We booked ourselves on an Air Canada flight that would get us in well before our interview, and we landed at Montreal's Dorval

International Airport right on schedule. Gloria Estefan was performing that night, so our meeting time was set for 1:30. I couldn't wait to meet her.

Gloria Estefan is one of the best-selling musical artists of all time. She has been around for more than four decades and is the undisputed original queen of Latin pop music. To date she has released thirty-one albums, selling over one hundred million records worldwide. Her band was originally known as Miami Sound Machine, but all albums after 1989's Cuts Both Ways have been credited to Gloria alone.

She was currently on tour promoting her new album, *Into the Light*. Most of the album was a reflection on her recovery from the spinal injury she suffered when a truck collided with her tour bus during a snowstorm in Pennsylvania.

As we took a taxi from the airport to our hotel, a sense of excitement filled me, mixed with some anxiety and urgency I could not shake. It was all I could do to take in the view. I was anxious to reach the hotel so that I could prepare for the interview; this was my opportunity to ask Gloria what she had overcome during her recovery and what it took to bring her to where she was today. Glen Baxter, the field producer with me, was nowhere near as excited as I was.

"Can you believe that we're actually here?" I asked Glen, the exhilaration obvious in my tone.

"We hardly had time to think while up there before we were landing."

The airplane ride had been very short. We'd been in the air about fifty minutes.

"Yes, I suppose it was a short trip. But we're here! And to think in mere hours I'll be talking one-on-one with Latin's queen of pop! Are you ready for all of this?"

Glen was a laid back kind of guy. He was tall, I'd guess close to six feet, with ginger red hair. There was something very attractive about his overall makeup, and he had a smooth way about him, a real charismatic appeal; a person would never feel out of sorts in his presence.

"You really shock me sometimes," I added. "We are preparing to meet an international superstar, and you're stuck on the time we didn't spend up in the air. How do you explain that?"

"Well Wendy, I guess all my time as a field producer with YTV is catching up with me," he said. "I am simply not as impressed by the job as I once was, or by the people I sometimes cross paths with."

Pulling up to the hotel had me a little out of sorts. The taxi driver had done a good job collapsing my wheelchair for the drive from the airport, but I wondered if he would reassemble it as easily – and he did.

It seemed no time before we were registered and ushered to our rooms. Although it had been made clear I would need an accessible room, I was concerned that it would lack proper access. I was pleasantly surprised to find everything was accessible to the wheelchair. Immediately after getting to my room, I took out my notes to go over the questions I had prepared for the interview. Glen was quick to react.

"Wendy, the interview is scheduled for one thirty this afternoon. You have more than enough time to prepare."

"Oh I suppose you're right," I agreed. "We could take in the sights. I know I'd like to try an order of poutine. I'm told there's no better place to have it but here in Montreal where it originated!"

"As a one time resident of Montreal I can honestly say the poutine served here does surpass what you find in Toronto," Glen confirmed. "I believe I'll join you in that indulgence."

Although I was slightly preoccupied with the upcoming interview, we made our way out of the hotel and through the streets of the Old Port of Montreal. The scenery was breathtaking, and the weather was certainly on our side. We walked along the boardwalk, taking in all the boats docked at port before indulging in our takeout order of poutine at 9:30 in the morning. There was little doubt that it was far superior to anything I had tasted back home. We stayed out for about an hour and a half – much of it spent people watching – before finding our way back to the hotel. There was a definite sense of style to the people of Montreal, their dress, their presence in general. It was like a trip to Europe; the mood, the language, the overall culture. I was taken in by it all.

Back at the hotel, I freshened up for the big moment, all the while going over in my mind the questions I would ask Gloria. The sense of anticipation was overwhelming. It seemed no time at all before Glen was outside my hotel room door. We were ready to go over to the auditorium.

We entered through the side doors. There was a room assigned for the interview, and we were immediately met and escorted to the appropriate area. My nerves felt raw. All that I had been anticipating throughout the week was finally happening. Gloria entered the room with an air of confidence and strength.

"Hello, it's a pleasure to meet you," she said, shaking my hand. The strength of her grip was like nothing I had felt before – or would expect, given her short frame. She appeared much smaller than she did on stage; I guessed she stood all of five foot five, even in small heels. She was a compact size but appeared very solid; there was little doubt this woman worked out. She wore a black body-hugging mini dress with cut-out short sleeves. Her hair was long, well past her shoulders, with a definite curl or wave to it. I immediately wondered if the curl was natural or permanent. Either way, she was very well put together.

"Hello Gloria, I'm Wendy here with YTV, Canada! So glad you've found the time to meet with me," I said. "Sorry we were unable to meet in Toronto prior to your concert last week. I'm not sure if you've read the reviews?"

"No, I don't make the reviews my business," she replied. "My husband, Emilio, reads the reviews. Things work much better that way."

"Then I hope he shared how great they were, Gloria. The Toronto audience really loved your concert," I said.

"Yes, yes, he did say they were pleased."

I wanted to speak to her about the accident and her recovery from her injuries.

"And how are you feeling, Gloria? You've overcome such a setback. How does it feel to perform now, after all you've been through?"

"It's all been a process that I've dedicated myself to. My recovery has been a godsend. That was not a fun night [the night of the accident]. Cognitively, it's all been a very spiritual experience."

"Really Gloria, many would be angry that something like that would happen. Can you elaborate?"

"Well Wendy, I wouldn't change what has happened. It's made me live my life in a much richer way. I feel a deeper connection with my fans. We at times go through life feeling an invincibility, a sense that no harm can come. The accident has changed all of that."

"You said it was a very spiritual experience. What did you mean by that?"

"I definitely learned the power of prayer, being raised Catholic in school. In fact, I felt people's prayers. It was amazing and I used it when recuperating. I did a lot of meditation and visualization of the nerves reconnecting. It was all an incredibly moving experience and has definitely strengthened my faith in God."

"Did family play a significant part in your recovery?"

"Emilio was definitely my rock. He saw us through all of it, most notably throughout the initial stages of recovery. I was in no position to watch over the family as I once had."

"How difficult was that?" I asked

"Those were some very challenging times. My many roles felt stripped from me. It was through my recovery that life was put into perspective. Many of the lyrics on this album reflect that."

"Your album's title, *Into the Light* – I'm assuming it represents where you find yourself today?"

"Absolutely. I saw some very dark days while recovering, but each day became a little brighter as I worked toward my recovery."

Just then we were interrupted. A radio station was there and ready to broadcast live with Gloria. Our interview was brought to a halt.

"In closing, what's the one message you would like to send to your fans?" I asked her.

"I would say it is to always believe in yourself, regardless of the darkness you might find yourself in. There is always a way out. It comes down to believing in yourself, and through the grace of God you will see better days."

"Well now, that was certainly well put. I know our viewers will be moved by this, Gloria," I added.

"Okay then, it appears I have a radio station awaiting me!"

And in a flash she was gone. All the anticipation suddenly lifted, and we had the material we wanted.

In a flash the interview was all over, but not the journey I had taken. What seemed a lifetime had in fact been a five-year span of tenacious efforts in my quest to deliver a better understanding of the physically challenged population. I had set out on a mission to expose and better educate the able-bodied world on the abilities possessed by many who find themselves using a wheelchair. It seemed now my call was being answered on a global scale. Not only did I have the Miss Venus International Pageant under my belt, taking home the Contestants' Choice Award, but I had collected a one-on-one interview with an American pop icon.

Although I remained in a wheelchair, my life was anything but limited! This feeling was never made more real than later that evening when I sat in the audience watching Gloria Estefan on stage.

Chapter 17: Front Page Challenge

Taking home the title of Miss Venus Swimwear added to my list of career accomplishments and resulted in an overwhelming amount of press. My win generated headlines such as "Overcoming Obstacles in Her Life" and "Paraplegic Model Winning Beauty Contest Hailed as Breakthrough." I was swept up in the magic. Radio and television interviews were requested by many of the local stations, the newspapers were calling, and my days were booked. I took it all in stride, talking myself through the stress of it all.

The last thing I expected was for the title to take me out of town for a guest appearance. It all began with a phone call from Rhona.

"Hello Wendy, how's my superstar?"

"Hey Rhona, doing fine. What's up?"

"I received a phone call from a CBC producer. Are you familiar with the television show, Front Page Challenge?"

"Somewhat, why?" I knew the show, but had never seen it.

"Well the show's producer, David Kines, wants you to be a guest on the program."

Rhona explained that this was a long-running game and interview show where famous Canadian journalists try to guess what news story the hidden guest is associated with. When the challenge is completed and the guest is revealed, the guest talks further with the panel about their news story.

"There is a catch to this, Wendy, and one I think you'll be thrilled with. They're taping the show on the east coast, so you will be taking an all-expense-paid trip to Charlottetown, Prince Edward Island."

I was thrilled to hear the taping would take place on Prince Edward Island, where my family's roots were and where friends were living who could perhaps attend the taping. There was also a one-time serious boyfriend, Robert Duffy, whom I had dated in Toronto for more than two years. He had since moved back to his PEI home town of Kinkora.

"It sounds like something I think I could do. What do you think, Rhona?" I asked.

"I think you will do great. You'll just be answering questions about the pageant. How could you go wrong?" she added.

"Do you mind if I think about it, talk it over with my family? When do you have to let them know?"

"They have asked that I let them know by Thursday, so you will have a few days to think about it."

"Thanks, Rhona. I'll talk it over with my mom and dad and get back to you."

"That's fine, Wendy, just don't let too many people know. You are to be the hidden guest."

I went down to the family room where my mom and dad were watching the evening news.

"I just had a call from Rhona. A CBC television producer has contacted her to ask about having me as a hidden guest on Front Page Challenge."

My parents were delighted with the idea that I would be a guest on a major TV show. My dad was a regular viewer and said that Pierre Berton had always been one of his favourite journalists. When I mentioned that the show would be taped in PEI, he brought up something I had been thinking of too.

"What about access, Wendy? Where will you be staying?"

"This is all something that will have to be worked out through Rhona. I told her it was a decision I would make after speaking with you both. The only way I would agree to this is if I'm provided with accessible accommodations. I do have apprehensions, since it is on the Island."

While Prince Edward Island was a wonderful place to visit, I knew it was far behind the other Canadian provinces on accessibility issues. I had made a number of visits to PEI during my relationship with Robert, only to be faced with frustration. Public parking and washrooms offered little access. Many of the homes were older in design and build, making them impossible to get around in.

After discussing it with my parents, I decided I would appear as a hidden guest on the legendary show. But not without first ensuring my accommodations were fully accessible. I made a point to call Rhona to express my concerns.

"Hey Rhona, it looks like it's a go for the show. My only concern is access in the hotel that I am to stay at. How many nights will I be there?"

"I have said that accepting the invitation would depend on the facilities available and the access they have to offer. I've made it clear that any issues limiting your access would call the whole deal off. The hotel they're suggesting is the Canadian Pacific Hotel, and you'll be there for two nights."

I was so happy that Rhona understood my circumstances and was dealing with the arrangements. Two nights would not take me outside my comfort zone too much and sounded very manageable. I told her to go ahead and accept the offer.

For the rest of the evening, my mind was consumed by the appearance I was going to make. I was not yet sure what I would wear on the show or what questions might be asked. I decided there was little to be gained by trying to guess what to expect. Instead I focused on the people I would have the pleasure of seeing back in PEI. There would be cousins to get in touch with, and perhaps tickets to reserve.

And thoughts swirled through my head about how far I had come.

They were almost like flashbacks of me back at Toronto Western Hospital wondering what would become of my life, how I would continue, and what would be my ultimate fate. There were no clues back then as to where I would eventually find myself. I had come through so much with few preconceived notions of exactly how my life would unfold, with little hope at times. Much of my future had been in question, but not anymore. I was moving forward faster than I could have anticipated, with doors opening that allowed me to fulfill the goals I had set out to achieve. My efforts had thrown me into the spotlight. I was showing others that a split second could put anyone in a wheelchair, and hopefully I was now demonstrating the abilities of the person in that wheelchair, taking the focus off the disability and placing it on the individual. That it would not only be their ability that would move them forward, but society's willingness to see beyond the wheelchair. It would all begin with an open mind and the opportunity. All that I was now achieving had come through the initial opportunity, someone willing to give me the chance, someone willing to see change, willing to move past the limiting notion of disability. While there was still a long way to go in the larger realm – access, jobs, transportation – I was definitely exposing the issue publicly. Mainstreaming the physically challenged was what I hoped for: an inclusive society that did not discriminate or exclude.

***

Nearly a month after I first learned about my Front Page Challenge appearance, my trip to Prince Edward Island was scheduled. I was thrilled to see the event finally arrive. My ticket on Air Canada was provided through CBC Television.

At Pearson Airport, I approached the check-in desk with my father. To my surprise, the airline was fully aware of my arrival.

"Hello Miss Murphy, we've been expecting you," the ticket agent said as I prepared to hand her my ticket.

When flying, people in wheelchairs are usually asked to be the first on the aircraft. I no longer abide by that rule, and here's why: On two occasions they have put me on the aircraft long before the rest of the passengers are boarded. By the time the flight took off, I needed to use the washroom. This meant that two airline attendants had to carry me to the lavatory. So I no longer allow them to board me first. Also, when I do approach the gate, I am sure that my bladder is thoroughly emptied.

The passengers were ready to board the aircraft at the time I approached the gate, making the boarding process as smooth as silk.

"If you'll take your carry-on bag, you can follow me down to the boarding gate," said the boarding agent.

We then proceeded from the airport doors onto the boarding ramp and down to the doors of the aircraft. It was there that I transferred onto the straight-back chair, leaving my wheelchair to be placed in the belly of the aircraft. I was then pulled backwards onto the aircraft and carefully down the aisle to my seat.

The flight was pleasant, with a younger mother and her five-year-old child sharing the two seats beside me. Sharon and her daughter, Ainsley, were from the Island and had spent the week with family that had uprooted themselves to the big city of Toronto.

Departing the aircraft was a similar process. My wheelchair was brought up to the doors of the airplane before they brought in the straight-back chair to assist me off the aircraft and onto the wheelchair.

As I entered the terminal I was greeted by a fellow who I assumed was the show's producer. "Wendy Murphy, Dave Kines. What can I say, other than we're thrilled to have you on board with us." He seemed excited that I had finally made it to Charlottetown.

"Hi Dave, and nice to finally put a face to the name," I replied. "Rhona mentioned you often while we were finalizing all the details."

We wasted no time in collecting my luggage and then headed to the car that was waiting for us. We continued our discussion as we drove.

"Your accomplishment is to be commended, Wendy. I respect what you are doing and the cause you represent."

I knew Dave was referring to my ongoing attempts to expose the issue of disability, getting it out there in any way I could. "I appreciate your commendation, but I don't see it as such a great feat. The universe appears to be on my side through it all."

"I have a first-hand understanding of the many obstacles you can face trying to get around in a wheelchair. My cousin was in a serious motorcycle accident five years ago. He's been in a wheelchair ever since. He's been great at adapting, and I know attitude has had a big role to play in it. He's since married and has two children. It seems he couldn't be happier."

"Moving forward is always key in recovery I've learned, and it sounds like your cousin has accomplished that. How old are his children?" I asked.

"They're both toddlers, one-and-a-half and three years old. Samantha and Alexia and are the apple of their father's eye."

"He sounds like a very lucky man," I added.

The drive from the airport to the CP Prince Edward Hotel was not long. I could not help wondering what accessibility challenges I might have to face. I was a little preoccupied thinking the hotel might not be as accessible as we had been told.

This was an issue I faced often when I was unsure about facilities I planned to visit, so I made enquiries. I was sometimes disappointed to find the facilities were not fully accessible at all. Would this be the case here?

It was now early evening. As soon as we arrived at the hotel, Dave made his way inside to find the best way for me to enter. It turned out that there was a ramp at the side of the hotel that would offer me full access into the building. Dave went back out to the car to retrieve my luggage and wheelchair. I then got myself onto the wheelchair before I headed to the ramp.

The hotel definitely offered access, with most of the rooms fully modified. "I'm thrilled to see the hotel can fully accommodate the wheelchair, Dave. I have no concerns about access. What time is the taping? What do I have to do while I'm here?" I asked

"Taping will take place tomorrow evening in the theatre of the Confederation Centre of the Arts. I estimate the night to go at least two full hours for the taping, with cocktails and finger foods to be served afterwards."

"I do have family and friends here on the Island that I would like to contact," I explained. "My Aunt Dorothy and cousin Carla have already gotten their tickets for the show. Not to worry, they've all been warned not to talk about my appearance. They understand that it's a mystery and meant to stay that way."

"I haven't mentioned the complimentary tickets!" said Dave. "You are entitled to two tickets for the taping of the show. Is there anyone else you'd like to invite?"

With my relatives already coming to the show, I wondered whether St. Clair and Clara Duffy, my former boyfriend Robert's parents, would attend the taping.

"That just may be a possibility, Dave. Leave it with me and I will let you know."

After Dave left, I grabbed a telephone book in my room and after looking Robert's parents up I gave them a call. I immediately recognized the voice of Robert's mother Clara.

"Hi Clara, it's Wendy ... Wendy Murphy from Toronto. How are you?" I asked.

"I'm great, Wendy, and so nice to hear from you. Where are you calling from?"

"Believe it or not, Clara, I am calling from Charlottetown. I'm on the Island."

I explained to her that I was there to tape Front Page Challenge. "The producer has just offered me two complimentary tickets and my aunts have already purchased theirs. If you and St. Clair are free tomorrow night and would like to see the taping you are both welcome to come as my guests."

"If you have tickets for us, we'd love to be part of the evening."

"That's great, Clara. I'm thrilled you will both be coming, it's been a while."

I immediately called Dave to let him know the tickets would be used by two guests.

Robert's family had been wonderful throughout our relationship. My visits to Prince Edward Island were always met with open arms and open doors by all of them. I would stay in their home while there and although it was not fully accessible, I would stay on the main level and talk for hours with his dad. He ran Duffy's Construction and was often at home directing the crew of workers.

I slept well in the Prince Edward Hotel that night. I figured it was all the travel and excitement. Dave had told me that a car would be by to pick me up no later than two-thirty the following afternoon. I would have a brief visit to makeup before taping would begin.

I dressed for the evening in a bright red chiffon blouse and black cigarette pant. I also decided to wear the black bolero hat that I had worn in the pageant.

I was pleasantly surprised to see Dave come to pick me up and take me to the theatre.

"Hello there," I called immediately after seeing him. "What a nice surprise to see you."

"I figured it would be easier all round," he said, "since I've had some experience collapsing the wheelchair and placing it into the trunk of the car. A more seamless transition. I'm hoping you're well rested and ready to go."

"I had a great sleep and spent most of the day wondering what would happen to me during the taping. It's been weeks of anticipation. I'll be glad to put it all behind me," I added.

When we arrived at the theatre I was immediately impressed with the accessibility that I saw. I followed Dave into the building and directly into makeup. The room was quite large and very well lit. There was no one there except the makeup artist.

"Hello Tess," said Dave. "This is Wendy, who'll be taping second this evening. Powder her up for the cameras," he instructed.

It was not until I was guided into the green room that I realized the extent of my appearance on the show. There were a number of people already comfortable in the room, including Robert Stanfield, seventeenth premier of Nova Scotia and leader of the Progressive Conservative Party, Sheila Copps, one of Canada's foremost female politicians, and Joyce Milgaard, who worked for twelve years to prove her son David's wrongful conviction for murder. I was honoured to be among such a recognized group.

"I am pleased to have you all here and ready for the taping," Dave announced after I joined the group. "It appears we're on time, so two hours should do it. We have a packed theatre out there and I am confident you'll all do a great job."

Not long after his announcement Dave came over to me with some news.

"Wendy we are trying something different with your segment of the show. I hope you're not disappointed by the change in plans, but there really is no other choice."

He told me I would not be hidden during my segment. The theatre had a winding staircase for the secret guests to climb, with a seat for them above and behind the panel. This would ensure their identity remained concealed while they were being questioned by the panelists.

But I would not be able to get up the stairs. I would have to be on the same level as the panelists, and they would be able to see me.

"That will work for me, Dave," I replied.

Still, I wondered if the panel would guess my headline.

After learning about my position on stage I regrouped with the other guests. I was excited that Robert Stanfield was there; Mike McInnis, my uncle's father always spoke so highly of him and his political views. I knew he would be proud to see me as part of the production. Sheila Copps was a Liberal MP; I had heard about her from my father, who was a staunch Conservative Party supporter. Shortly after I got back to the group, Dave briefed us about what was happening out in the theatre.

"The panelists have taken their place in the theatre and I think we are just about ready to begin taping. Fred Davis will be moderating this evening and the panel will include Pierre Berton, Betty Kennedy, Gordon Sinclair, and Jack Webster. We have a packed house. Does anyone have any questions?"

Because I would be joining the panelists on stage, it was decided that my story would be moved to first taping. Like the set of Street Legal, there were many light cables and cords we had to get the wheelchair over before I was able to enter the stage through a side entrance.

I was not fully prepared for what awaited me, the bright lights, crowds of people and the audience's applause. I looked to my left and was greeted with a warm and encouraging smile from Pierre Berton, who sat behind a long desk with the other panelists but was closest to me. The applause seemed to go on forever before Fred Davis formally addressed me.

"Good evening, first contestant, and welcome to Front Page Challenge. Your circumstances have given our panelists an advantage, you will not be concealed from them this evening, let us see how they'll do. Now then, Pierre, you will start with the questions."

"Well, I have definitely seen you in the media," was how he began.

"Did your story have legal ramifications?"

"No," I answered.

"Is this a happy story?"

"Yes."

"Is this a politically driven story?"

"No."

At that point, questions moved over to Betty Kennedy.

"Are you a doctor, lawyer, or teacher of some kind?"

"No," again, was my response.

"Does your headline in any away involve your work, or professional life?"

This is where I was a little confused about how to answer. The pageant was by no means a profession I had taken up, although it did fall into my modelling career. After receiving advice from Fred Davis I answered the question.

"Yes."

"Are you in the political realm at all?"

"No."

Wow, I thought. They are really perplexed.

The questions would now come from Gordon Sinclair.

"Are you a professional athlete, involved in the Paralympics?" he asked.

"No," was my response.

"Are you a wife?"

"No."

"Are you a mother?"

"No."

"Is your story in any way affiliated with a win of some kind?"

Finally, a second yes, I thought.

"Yes."

"Have you won a lottery, some type of ticket you purchased that has paid off?"

"No," I responded.

Jack Webster was now up for questions.

"Do you reside in the province of Ontario?"

"Yes."

"Is this win monetary?"

I was again, unsure of how to answer the question. I did receive prizes. With the guidance of Fred Davis, I answered, "Yes."

The questions then went back to Pierre Berton and made their way back around to each of the panelists, giving them all one more chance with their questions. After that, their time ran out. They were unable to figure out my headline. Fred Davis then took over the stage.

"The headline was 'Pageant Hopeful Doesn't Sit Around.' Ladies and gentlemen, please join me in welcoming, Miss Wendy Murphy."

The applause and whistles roared through the theatre, and I was moved by the audience's reaction. It was at that time that the panelists were offered the opportunity to question me once again, knowing now how I had made the news.

They began once again with Pierre Berton.

"Well Wendy, you appear to be quite a courageous young lady. Were you at all surprised with your win at this pageant, and how do you believe society has changed where disabilities are concerned?"

"Well Mr. Berton, I have definitely witnessed change in attitudes. I do not believe I would be on this stage tonight if it weren't for those changes, although there's always room for improvement."

"And where could those improvements be made, Wendy?" he asked.

"Access is a big issue. Maintaining my independence is of the utmost importance in continually moving forward with my life. Not relying on others to help me up that curb, or to open that heavy door will alleviate my dependence. It's a liberating feeling."

Betty Kennedy then joined in.

"Wendy, are you trying to tell the world that you are intelligent, beautiful, and capable in every way?"

"I'm hoping to tell the world that we are here, and we aren't going away. The more we are seen – I'm referring to the disabled population – the more opportunities will advance for us and access will eventually improve. We are all capable of contributing, giving back to society. We are just looking for the opportunities to do so."

"What about the other girls, how did they react to your participation?" Gordon Sinclair asked.

"The girls were fabulous in both competitions. In fact, I took home the Contestants' Choice Award from the international competition. That just about sums it all up!" I replied.

Jack Webster then, on behalf of all the panelists, wished me continued success.

It seemed like a flash and it was over. I had been anticipating the taping of the show for more than a month and just like that, it was done. I could now relax and enjoy the rest of the evening. But not without realizing all that I was able to get across to the panel regarding disability, and how we played a part in today's society. If we were no longer limited by attitudes, we could all make our mark in this world.

Chapter 18: The Big Move

I remained thrilled with the ongoing support of my family, but there came a point when I felt ready to test my independence. The idea of finding my own place to live became a tantalizing thought.

I knew there would be many things to consider if I were to take on the responsibility of living alone, access being a number-one priority. But there were also a number of other issues. Living with my family, I always had someone watching my back. If I needed anything I couldn't reach, for example, simply calling out to someone quickly solved my dilemma. Any time I needed help there were always ways around the situation. Living alone would put a whole new spin on things. At times I wondered if going solo was really something I really wanted to do. My concerns also surrounded our family home, which had been purchased and modified especially to accommodate my needs. Many of the changes could have been avoided if I hadn't decided I would join the family after my discharge from Lyndhurst. I couldn't help but feel a little guilty. One afternoon I shared my aspirations as well as my concerns with my mom and dad.

"Mom, Dad ... I believe I am ready for a change."

"Just what kind of change did you have in mind?" my mother asked.

"Big change actually. After a lot of thought and serious consideration I'm contemplating moving out on my own."

"What's brought this on?" my father asked.

"I can assure you both this is not a whimsical notion, but something I have put some great thought toward before coming to you with it. Before we go any further I want you both to know the depths of my gratitude to you for the support you've shown since the accident. I don't think I would have ever come this far without you. Being on my own now just feels like the next step for me."

My father was quick to jump in.

"We would not have done anything differently if the situation was to happen again. We are amazed at the strength you've shown through all of this, Wendy. We know you've seen some tremendously difficult times while trying to overcome your challenges, and just know how proud we are of you, dear."

"We'll definitely support you in any choice you make about your living arrangements, Wendy. You've come a long way," my mom added.

Any doubts that I had regarding the backing I might or might not receive from my parents evaporated as the discussion evolved.

"You both have no idea how much this means to me, the relief I'm feeling now that the topic is on the table for discussion. It's been on my mind for a while now. I'm forever grateful to you both."

My mother's eyes swelled with tears before responding.

"You are grateful?" There was a slight pause as she composed herself. "What can we really say other than you've proven to be a very determined young lady through all of this, and we are constantly surprised by your strength and perseverance. Wendy, you have proven to us all that challenges, regardless of their nature, can be overcome."

"This would certainly be a change for you, living on your own," she added, "but if it's something you feel ready for, we are here to support you, dear."

"That's what I hoped to hear, Mom."

After giving their approval, my parents suggested that I get in touch with Sean Yeates, a real estate agent with years of experience, who was also a family friend. My parents felt that bringing him on board would make the search for a rental property much easier. I wasted no time in contacting him.

"Hello Sean, Wendy Murphy here. Pauline and Gerald's daughter."

"Oh yes, Wendy, how can I help you?"

"I have decided that I might be ready to live on my own. I am interested in looking at some rental properties."

We discussed a few possible locations before setting up a time to meet the following day. The possibility of finding my own place to live was now a focus, and I could hardly get it out of my mind. It was exciting to think about the actual hunt for a new place, and moving in and decorating.

Early the next day I drove into Sean's driveway with nothing but positive thoughts filling my mind.

He was already standing there, awaiting my arrival.

"Are we all ready for a day of sightseeing?" Sean asked.

"Sounds good to me!" I was really anxious to be getting on with the adventure.

"I figured we would start our search in the Mississauga area, somewhere close to your current community. After all, this is where you will find yourself spending most of your time, with the majority of your friends currently located close by.

"I've chosen three condominiums to see first. Given your intention to rent, we won't be considering any units that require out-of-pocket modifications. This might limit the number of available units, but we'll get a better idea of our options more when we are actively looking."

I hadn't thought about the need for modifications, but I hope we'd know more after we looked through a couple of the possibilities.

Sean did the driving with me as the passenger. We'd decided it would be easier to map our way around the city with him behind the wheel.

At the first condominium, I was immediately impressed with the exterior. The building had fifteen floors, and the unit I was seeing was on the fourth floor.

However, as Sean and I entered the condominium, there was not much more to be impressed about. I found the unit to be small and the broadloom very dark, closing the space in.

We explored the living room, dining room, and kitchen. It was modest in size, and dated in decor. Unimpressed by the initial impression we left the unit.

184 Wendy Murphy's Law

"Now don't get discouraged, Wendy," Sean insisted as we went back out to his car. "You are just beginning your journey in the rental market. We'll have this down to a science in no time."

The second unit for rent impressed me much more. While the exterior of the building didn't offer much in style or structure, the unit was very impressive. It had wall-to-wall carpet once again, but this time in a light beige tone. This unit also had a balcony. After seeing the kitchen, I was growing more attached to the layout. Feeling positive I headed into the bedroom to see if this could be the unit for me. Once again, I was impressed.

My optimism was dashed however with a visit to the washroom. I could barely make my way past the doorway with very limited clearance for the wheelchair once I was through the door.

Considering the washroom problem it didn't look like this unit would be my new home either.

"Are we sure this unit won't work?" I asked Sean. "There appears to be so much that's right about it."

"Wendy, there's no way this washroom will facilitate you or the wheelchair, and we're not about to invest money into modifying a unit you plan on renting."

I knew he was right but I was thoroughly disappointed.

One thing we had learned was that we should begin any inspection with the washrooms to ensure the facilities would be wheelchair accessible.

The third and final suite we saw did little to entice either of us. In fact, I had been so impressed by the previous unit I was unable to think of anything but it.

We entered the unit through the living room.

"I'm sorry, Sean, but I can't help thinking about the last unit we looked at. It was such a well-laid-out floor plan. If it wasn't for that damned bathroom I would be signing papers as we speak."

"I know you were taken by that last unit, Wendy. It's important not to give up. There's a unit waiting, with your name all over it, I can feel it. What do you say we call this a day and make another try tomorrow?"

"I think you might be right."

After returning home, I gave myself time to reflect on the day. It was hard to believe I was actually out shopping for a rental unit, a new place to live independently of my family. I was in awe at how far I had actually come since those desperate days at Toronto Western Hospital.

Sean and I resumed our search the following day, although this time with a much better system in place: in any place we saw, we would head directly for the bathroom. It made sense to eliminate those that did not offer me access. From there, we would move on to the kitchen to see if it would offer a moderate amount of access without renovations.

After venturing in and out of what seemed to be an endless array of possible rentals, we ended up in a penthouse unit. Of course I began with a visit to the bathroom.

"Okay Sean, this place is not a contender. This bathroom would never accommodate me fully."

"Hold on a second, Wendy. I'm here, in the master bedroom." His voice echoed. "Come in here for a second."

I entered into a massive room complete with a bay window. Sean was pointing into the en suite bathroom. I was speechless. The floors were done in a bone coloured marble with gold-toned sink, toilet, and bathtub. The tub was surrounded by mirrors and I wheeled into it with ease before making a full turn of my wheelchair and referring back to Sean.

"Well," I said, pleasantly surprised, "let's look at the rest."

Making our way out of the master bedroom I closely examined the rest of the condominium and its features. This could, after all, be the place I would call home.

As we headed back up the hallway, I revisited what would be the spare bathroom if I decided to take the unit. There was a second bedroom across from it. Back at the front door we looked into the living room, dining room, and solarium. The wall-to-wall carpet was a very light beige tone and warmed the whole living space. From the dining room we made our way into the kitchen, which had a balcony and an entrance into the solarium. I was absolutely thrilled with the unit. This was the one!

"We have to move fast on this one, Sean, I don't want to lose it."

We raced back to the real estate office to prepare the paperwork. To increase my chances of being accepted for the rental property, we included my résumé and a few of my Bay Department Store flyers.

I took possession of the condominium at Twenty Cherrytree Drive almost immediately.

I resided there for a little more than eight years.

Chapter 19: Sights Set on Television

With YTV and a number of guest appearances on various television shows under my belt, and as a part-time student at Ryerson University in the Radio and Television Arts course, I was now ready to move forward with my ultimate goal of becoming a television personality. City TV was where I had set my sights. I had been a guest on a number of the station's programs including Breakfast Television, Fashion Television, and Movie Television. I had also noticed that minorities and differently abled people were represented through the station's programming. A wheelchair, however, was not yet in their mix.

There were several routes to take, and a demo tape was necessary if I wanted to secure an on-air position. A demo tape is a product of your on-air abilities, much like a résumé, with short segments taken from the full body of your work. It also gives a potential employer an opportunity to see if the camera agrees with you. For some people, the camera is their best friend, so it is difficult for them to look bad through the eye of the lens. Others can take a horrible picture or are not as favoured by the camera lens. The tape should not be long, maybe five or six minutes in length depending on its purpose, and should offer a variety of one's work. I was hoping Phyllis Newman, a TV producer and editor, would work on my demo tape, and it all began with a phone call.

"Hello Phyl, it's Wendy Murphy calling. Hope all is well and wonder what you're up to."

"Hey there Wendy, what a nice surprise, it's been a while. I'm doing great! Still busy at Sleeping Giant productions, doing some editing and producing there. Why, what's up?" she asked.

"I'm hoping to put a demo tape together and I can think of no one better to help me produce it than you, that's if you have the time and are game for it."

"What time frame are we looking at? Is there a deadline for this?"

"Nothing pressing but I would like to see it put together ASAP. What kind of time can you give me?" I asked.

"I could certainly fit you in. What do you hope to include in the demo? What do I have to work with, Wendy?"

"My segments on Street Noise are a given. I would like to get a little creative, include the various talk shows I have been a guest on over the course of my success, perhaps include my skiing for CTV sports, and we can't forget my appearance on Front Page Challenge. That is a national production and takes in a vast audience. What do you say we meet up and talk more about this project? Please tell me you're willing to work with me on this."

Phyllis said she was willing, although she was only available on weekends.

"Can we hope to get started this coming weekend?" I asked.

"Yes, this weekend should be fine. Do you have this material on VHS tapes with a time code? This would allow me to paper-edit the work you'd like to see on the tape prior to getting into the editing bay. We could save a lot of time and money going that route."

"That's a great idea, Phyllis, thanks for suggesting it. I'll work on getting the material dubbed over from Beta format to VHS. I should have that for you later this week."

I said goodbye to Phyllis; now with my demo tape soon to be produced, it was time to work on my connections. There were a number of press clippings, some dating back to the time I began with Rhona and her agency. There were also press stories profiling me alone, and my accomplishments while working through the Star Tracks Talent Agency, including a breakthrough with The Bay when they used physically challenged models in their flyers and catalogues, modelling with Canadian designer Franco Mirabelli, and of course my victory at the Miss Venus Swimwear Toronto Pageant. I began distributing my résumé and the press kit I had prepared to those I felt could facilitate my efforts in finding a place at City TV's family of stations and television programs. There were a number to choose from, including the City TV newsroom, MuchMusic, and the weekly show, Fashion Television, hosted by Jeannie Becker, whom I had grown to know well since venturing into modelling.

I sent both Jeannie Becker and the producer of Fashion Television, Jay Levine, a personal package. Jay responded with a phone call.

"Hello Wendy, this is Jay Levine calling. You dropped off a package for me looking for a position in the Fashion Television family."

"Hello Jay, thank you so much for the phone call."

"Wendy, unfortunately there is nothing available here at the show at present but I wanted to thank you for your interest in joining us. I was impressed with the package you put together and wanted to let you know I passed it on to Moses Znaimer, the Executive Producer of nearly everything that goes on here at 299 Queen Street West. He's a very innovative man and would appreciate the mission you've set out on."

"I want to thank you so much for the gesture, Jay. I will definitely follow up with him."

Hanging up the telephone I was touched by his insightful generosity. I was sure he received countless résumés, considering the show's international audience. The time and effort he took to pass on the package I forwarded showed a real touch of class. I decided I would follow up with the press package he had forwarded to Mr. Znaimer with my demo tape, when the work was completed.

I went into the kitchen and ran my plan past my mother.

"I just might get somewhere professionally this weekend. I'll be working on a demo tape that will hopefully help me find work as an on air contributor with City TV."

"That's a tall order, Wendy, but I am sure you can manage it judging by your success so far."

"That's good to hear because my mind is made up. That's the career path I'll be following. I know it's a pretty bold statement to make since I am in a wheelchair."

"A fact that has not held you back from much the past few years," said my mother. "You know, Wendy, we have always supported your efforts. Why would you think that would end now, after all the success you've achieved? It's just important that you keep things in perspective. You've come a long way since your injury, but let's not lose sight of all that's truly important in life."

It was a very busy week, and a time of reflection. Phyllis had asked for all my potential television work to be transferred onto VHS tapes, and when I began collecting the work I had done, there was quite a lot to choose from. My YTV work aside, winning the pageant had brought me clear across country on the talk show circuit. Breakfast Television, Front Page Challenge, and the Dini Petty Show here in Canada, Sally Jessy Raphael in New York City, and the Carol and Marilyn Show in Los Angeles, California.

My efforts to publicize the issue of disability are definitely making their mark, but will this continue? I wondered. What would be the chances that I could find a place within the broadcasting industry for me and my wheelchair? While society appeared ready for an inclusive norm in advertising, was the broadcasting world also ready for this transition? After much thought I decided the only real way to answer my questions was to just go for it, to put all of my energy and efforts into the task of finding employment within the broadcasting industry. I had succeeded in my other attempts to get the message out and perhaps, with a little effort, something substantial could come of this too. I decided that I owed it to myself to give this venture my all, regardless of the barriers I might face. It was a change in attitudes that I was working to achieve, and finding my way through the obstacles would be the only way to achieve my goal of an on-air position. This was something I definitely had to pursue.

I woke early the morning I was to meet Phyllis at Stonehenge Productions, a facility located in downtown Toronto. I was a little concerned that the building would not be fully accessible, a problem

I had run into many times when venturing into the city, with parts of the downtown area being older and building structures not built according to new building codes. I figured between the two of us we could solve any problems that might appear. There would also be an editor by the name of Jamie, who Phyllis assured me would be there to use his muscles if they were in any way needed.

The facility was located on a one-way downtown street, not an easy place to find your way to. There was very limited parking. I was pleased to see Phyllis as I searched for a parking spot.

"Hey there Phyl! Glad to see we've made it!" I yelled out to her while pulling down the street. "I just might need a hand parking this baby."

Parking when driving with hand controls is always a challenge, but finding my way into this spot was definitely going to be a test. Eventually, I allowed Phyllis to park the car. My car can be driven by anyone licenced to drive. The hand controls are attached to the gas and brake pedals and do not prohibit someone using their feet or force them to use the hand controls.

Parking the car was just the beginning of our challenges. We were both disappointed to find three stairs into the Stonehenge Production facilities, where Jamie's assistance was a must. It all began with a simple introduction.

"Wendy, I'm pleased to introduce you to our man of the hour, Jamie. He'll be in charge of editing this project," Phyllis declared.

"In that case the pleasure is all mine," I responded. "Good morning, Jamie, I'm looking forward to working with you. Phyllis has spoken highly of you."

"Don't put too much pressure on me ladies, it's too early in the morning," was Jamie's initial response. "Now how can I be of help?"

With Jamie lifting the back of the wheelchair and Phyllis at the front, they were able to hoist me up the few stairs at the front of the production facility. Once in, we all made our way into the editing bay where Phyllis took out her notes and I began passing the tapes over to Jamie. We were there to work, with the cost of the editing bay charged by the hour. The faster we could get this done, the better off I would be financially.

Phyllis wasted no time getting started.

"I thought we would start the opening with flashes of all your guest spots on the talk shows, with music playing in the background. We want to capture our audience – your potential employers – with punch, a form of action.

"From the opening I'd like to start with your piece from Movie Television. There are some great segments of you modelling with bright lights and a fan, fanning your hair. That sets the mood for what's next. You speak about wanting to move into broadcasting with your career, which would bring us to your work at YTV."

"Wow Phyl, you've thought this through well."

"From the Movie Television piece we'll then move on to the Dini Petty Show. I really like the way you clearly stated your full intentions in going public with your mission. How you hope to promote the disabled through your modelling, and that the timing is right to see all media producers more open to employing those with disabilities.

"You're very frank with your choice of words. You really got your point across with that talk with her. This will only reinforce your point to those you hope will hire you.

"From there I would go to Betty Kennedy and your Front Page Challenge clip, stating that you hope to remain stylish, sexy, and a woman in every way. That gets even more of your message across to the viewer," Phyllis concluded.

While Phyllis and I continued to discuss where how we would structure the tape, Jamie began going through the tapes I had brought. He was quick to react to them.

"Wow, Wendy, you've got some great visuals here. Look at you skiing! You've got some national attention going on. I'm sure all of this has been work for you."

"Why, thanks Jamie. Yes, it has been work, but the work has somehow found me since I journeyed out of my comfort zone and challenged the advertisers. I feel very passionate about exposing the issue of disability, promoting it to the general public. The disabled community needs a voice, a role model right now. If I can be that voice then my mission is accomplished. Finding a career in mainstream television is my new goal now."

"Well, if the material you've collected here today is a reflection of your determination," said Jamie, "I see you moving on to mainstream television with no problem. You've had some very impressive exposure, that I am sure will impress a few producers."

"Thank you again, Jamie, your encouragement means a lot. I guess it has been a successful run so far."

The day went well, with the three of us collaborating on the project, and the creative juices were definitely flowing. We were together for a good five hours of work. I was feeling much better about what I was setting out to accomplish after brainstorming with Jamie and Phyllis. I couldn't thank the two of them enough when we finally completed the demo tape; not for just the tape we had created together, but the physical efforts to get me into and out of the building.

After the long day spent with Phyllis and Jamie, there was much to do at home. My sister Kim and I were expecting guests for the evening. We decided on the gathering to celebrate the birthday of one of Kim's co-workers, Sharon Wilson. It would be an intimate gathering with no more than ten of us expected; beer and wine were to be served with pizza ordered later that night, before birthday cake. Sharon had been a close friend of Kim's for some time, like part of the family. I arrived home early evening to find Kim rushing around, preparing for our guests to arrive.

I decided I would not mention too much about my quest to move into broadcasting until things looked a little more promising. I didn't want the family to think I was setting my sights too high.

I set about preparing the den for the guests and made it to my room to get ready to greet the crowd. I couldn't help but think about the day I had spent with Jamie and Phyllis preparing my demo tape, going over the flow of the segments included and just how well they would represent me and my ultimate goal. I was definitely impressed with the work Phyllis had put into the project, and wondered how others would react when viewing the tape and the message we hoped to project. Was my goal actually achievable or a far-fetched ambition with little chance of flourishing?

It was no time before our guests began arriving, with Chris McPhee the first on board. Chris worked at Canadian Airlines with my sister Kim and Sharon Wilson. He lived close to us and was a frequent guest in our home. He was a very handsome young man with dirty blonde hair and blue coloured eyes. He stood very tall, I would guess six foot two with a solid build. There was no mistaking the friendship he seemed to share with my sister Kim, which the family would tease her about when we found the chance. Kim cared dearly for him as a friend, but she felt no romantic sparks.

"Hey there Chris, welcome. It's been a while," I said as he came through the front door.

"Hello there superstar, any trips to Hollywood planned yet?" Chris threw at me. "I saw another Bay flyer adorned with your presence. I'm thrilled to see things happening for you."

It was an acknowledgement I was often given by those who knew me. Many were thrilled to see my life in such a great place, given the physical challenges I faced. They were happy to see me making a mark for myself, following through with my convictions.

"Thanks Chris, I'm really enjoying the ride."

Next to arrive was Gina, who always had a way of making her presence be known, and never arrived empty handed.

"I come bearing gifts," she stated as I opened the front door to let her in. In one hand she had a six-pack of wine coolers, and in the other, a copy of the Bay flyer with me in it! "My mother has asked for an autograph," she said.

I could not help but appreciate their gestures and comments; in fact, they were reaffirming to me. They let me know that what I was doing was setting a precedent, offering inclusion into the general population for those using a wheelchair. We are here and not going away, I thought.

Only time would tell whether my ultimate goal of television reporter would come to fruition. It was a difficult industry for anyone to approach, let alone someone with a physical disability. But I was halfway there, with nothing stopping me now, and a demo tape prepared to take me through the fundamental stages.

Chapter 20: Making My Rounds

In the summer of 1993, I was driving home from Ryerson after a class called The On Camera Experience, and I once again took time to reflect on where I was in my life. I was making strides in my professional career, I was living independently, confident in my abilities, and I had a group of incredible friends. And of course Grania was forever in my thoughts. I wondered where we both might be if we had not been faced with such tragedy. I had little doubt my professional life would have unfolded more traditionally if I had continued working at Domtar. I now found myself in a more public role.

I started thinking about my plan for a more permanent and higher profile role at City TV. My demo tape was complete and I was hoping to meet City's co-founder and leader, Moses Znaimer. As if my thoughts had been read, I arrived home to find a message on my answering machine from Moses Znaimer's assistant, Carol Love, requesting a meeting. I returned the call immediately.

"Well, hello Wendy," said Carol, "and thank you for getting back to me. Jay Levine passed on your press kit to Moses and he would like a meeting with you. Would you be available next Thursday at around 2:00 p.m.?"

"Thursday at two it is. Thank you, Carol."

I hung up the phone feeling elated. I couldn't believe the meeting was going to happen so easily, and I had Jay Levine, the producer of Fashion Television, to thank. He'd said when we spoke that he had passed my press kit on to Moses Znaimer, which was obviously how I got the meeting. Elated or not, I decided I was hungry, so I made a sandwich while I imagined just how the meeting would unfold.

Moses was the mastermind behind much of the programming at City TV as well as the independent television stations that aired from their headquarters, such as MuchMusic and Bravo. A graduate of McGill University, Moses Znaimer's initiation into television began at CBC Television in Toronto, where he directed, produced, and hosted several programs from 1965 to 1969. Hoping to create a more dynamic television mix, he launched City TV, channel 79 (later 57), where he developed the concept of participatory or interactive TV, with no traditional studios and more of a storefront design. His ultimate goal was to create TV that reflected those watching it, and his stations went to great lengths to include many of the cultural, ethnic, and diverse programs and people in Toronto and throughout Canada. I knew my wheelchair would add to his eclectic mix.

I was delighted with all that was happening but I decided to keep my thoughts to myself for the time being, not wanting to draw too much attention to my goal of becoming a City TV television reporter. Many people I knew would feel I was grasping for the impossible given my circumstances, and I did not want to set myself up for disappointment among my peers. Besides, it was Friday afternoon, and the meeting was less than a week away; although I was bursting with excitement, this was a situation I would keep to myself – for now.

I managed to keep myself busy for the next week, and the day of my appointment to meet with Moses Znaimer arrived quickly. I woke early that morning, leaving myself lots of time to prepare for the meeting. After a long bath, I faced the question of what to wear. Because I had kept the news of the meeting to myself, I had eliminated any chance to solicit suggestions about what to wear to the big event. It was summer and my skin was tanned, so I decided on a cream-coloured sleeveless blouse with a tan pair of dress pants; colours that would complement my sun-kissed body and light blonde hair.

Never one to be late for appointments, I gave myself plenty of time to arrive at 299 Queen Street West. I had confirmed earlier that parking would be available, and a security guard accompanied me to Moses Znaimer's office, where I was greeted by his assistant, Carol Love.

"Good afternoon, Wendy. Glad to see you've made it."

"Thank you for making sure the parking was available, Carol. It made driving here possible."

"It was my pleasure. I've had a call from Moses and it seems he's running late. Make yourself comfortable in the sitting area. He should be around shortly."

After the anticipation of the meeting, my nerves were jangled with the thought of having to put things off any longer. I was now sitting in the office of a media icon, a man who through his vision and talent had changed the face of broadcasting. It had been a daring venture that many were waiting to see fail. But other cable stations followed: MuchMusic and Musique Plus (a venture based out of Montreal), both 24-hour music stations, the first of their kind. The longer I waited, the more nervous I felt. Although his disapproval wouldn't discourage me, I wondered what he would think of my aspirations to become an on-air personality. I had strong feelings about the need for a more diverse display of talent in television reporting, and I knew I would be a perfect fit for the job.

After about forty-five minutes, Mr. Znaimer finally arrived at the office.

"Hello Wendy, my sincere apologies for my tardiness. I was held up at my last meeting outside the office. Will you forgive me?"

He held both hands up toward his face as though he was praying for forgiveness, and I was touched by this seemingly sensitive display of character.

"Not a problem at all," I responded.

He was much more engaging than I had anticipated. As he was an astute businessman, I'd thought he would be taller, that his presence would command the room, but this didn't happen. Dressed in black, he had an alluring sense of mystery about him that I couldn't help but notice. He walked over to me with regal flair, offering his hand for a friendly handshake.

"It's a pleasure to meet you, Wendy. So glad we were able to make this meeting happen."

I was at a loss for words. I still wasn't sure exactly why I had been called to the meeting, so I simply let him know I was intrigued to be there.

"I was surprised to hear from your secretary," I added, "but thrilled with the call."

Moses then guided me into his office, a very large space that screamed character. He had a very long and well-organized desk. There were books stacked to one side and public broadcasting awards displayed at the opposite end. Below the vaulted ceilings, one wall was fully occupied with various career accomplishments, while another wall exhibited photographs of Moses with some very prominent people.

"So this is where Moses Znaimer lives, where the new age of television is brought to life. I must say I am impressed with the atmosphere you've created here," was my initial reaction. Moses was quick to respond.

"I'm glad to hear you are impressed. Many creative projects have been developed behind this closed door. Now tell me a little about Wendy Murphy."

"What would you like to know?"

"Well, what would you like to tell me?"

"I'm the middle child of three, I live in the west end of the city, and unlike most people, I hate pastries."

I thought I would throw a bit of humour in to the conversation, and Mr. Znaimer played along.

"Pastries? What else is on your hate list?"

"You first," I insisted.

"Okay, I hate being taken for granted."

"Most would agree with you there," I added.

I could feel Moses was trying to get to know me, while freeing the room of any tension or awkwardness.

"Well I'm sure you know that it was Jay Levine who passed on your press kit to me, which is why you are here today. I'm very impressed with your strength, Wendy, all that you've accomplished. I'm curious to know what makes you tick."

I decided to cut to the chase.

"As you've read, I was in a car accident, which put me in the wheelchair. But that has hardly stopped me. My mission is to expand exposure for the physically challenged population. I try to do this by highlighting abilities rather than disabilities."

"That is very commendable, Wendy. Just how do you intend to carry out your mission?" he asked.

"An on-air position would definitely be a promising start," I suggested.

Suddenly my mouth was very dry, a side effect of a medication I had to take. I could feel my lips sticking to my teeth. At that point Mr. Znaimer asked if I would like a drink of water, and I accepted his kind offer. While he made his way over to the mini bar to collect my drink, I decided it was time to add to the conversation.

"The people here at City TV do not 'tell' the news, they share it," I began. "There's a quality to their reporting that brings the viewer in, unlike any of the other news stations. I think Anne Mroczkowski, [who was the evening news anchor at that time] is a very dynamic woman. Some people I know are put off by her style, but I believe it's the strength she exudes through her on-camera work that sometimes threatens others."

Moses smiled endearingly while nodding his head yes. He walked over to his telephone, dialed an extension, and I heard, "Annie, are you busy? Can you come up to my office?"

I was flabbergasted. I felt like I was dreaming but knew that I wasn't. Here I was sitting in Moses Znaimer's office, about to meet Anne Mroczkowski!

It was not long before we heard a knock on the door.

"Come in," Moses called out.

I immediately turned to my right and watched Anne enter the office. She moved with grace and style as she walked over to Moses. He immediately referred to my press kit clippings on his desk before speaking.

"This is Wendy Murphy, Anne, and she's done some remarkable things with her life. She would like to get into television."

Turning to me, Anne approached me with her right arm extended, ready to shake hands.

"Why, hello Wendy, it's my pleasure to meet you."

"No, Anne, the pleasure is truly mine. I admire your work," I replied.

Anne's visit was brief but I was excited that I had actually met her. The mood in the room now became much more relaxed, I suddenly felt like I was sharing quality time with a friend.

"Tell me more about your family," Moses asked.

"As I mentioned earlier I am the middle child of three, an older sister Kim and younger brother Jeff," I explained. "My family have been instrumental in all that I've overcome. They've supported me through it all."

"One could only imagine. But you've made quite a remarkable recovery. Look what you have accomplished, and all while in a wheelchair."

Coming from him, the words meant a lot. My achievements resonated with me for a moment as I reflected, then I offered him my own insight.

"What I've learned over time is that it all comes down to perspective and how you choose to look at life. My rehabilitation has been a critical component in allowing me to move forward with my life. I believe we all have it in us to triumph, regardless of the circumstances. We must keep moving forward."

"I see you've brought a tape with you. Would that be your demo tape?"

"Yes, yes, it is," I replied offering it to him.

Moses took the tape and inserted it into the VCR player. When the tape ended Moses made his way around the desk and sat down next to me.

"What do you think of politics?"

"That would be a very touchy subject in our household. My father is a staunch conservative."

"What do you think of education?" he asked next.

"That would depend on what subject we were talking about."

"What about the weather?"

"I'm always happy when the sun's shining," I quickly added.

I knew now that he was trying to find a niche for me, trying to uncover a personal passion. Out of nowhere I hit his right leg with my left hand and asked, "How did Brona get her gig?" and he suddenly smiled broadly. I was talking about a Video Diary segment hosted by Brona Brown at that time, which aired on weekends. The segment highlighted personal milestones and community success stories.

"Brona has been with City TV for many years now, working behind the scenes," Moses explained. "She was looking for something more, so I resurrected the segment for her to host. The Video Diary is an old concept of community news that lets the general public become the star of the show."

"I think it's a brilliant concept, a great way to draw in your audience," I replied.

"Wendy, I have someone I would like you to meet," Moses stated suddenly. "The people downstairs in the newsroom are visionaries and run things their own way. I think it would be very advantageous for you to meet them."

I was prepared to follow through on any suggestion he had if it would bring me closer to my goal.

Moses went over to his desk and wrote down a name: Stephen Hurlbut, Director of News Programming.

"I'll speak to Stephen, give him some background on your situation. On-air positions are hard to come by Wendy, but let's see if we can make something work for you."

The meeting with Moses lasted for a little more than two and a half hours, a memory I hold dear to this day. It was a surreal experience. I went into the meeting not knowing what to expect from a man I had only read about, and I was pleasantly surprised. With his many years as a television icon, Moses welcomed me with no preconceived notions but a true sense of curiosity. He made the whole experience comfortable, opening up to me on many levels while I opened up to him. There was no ego and definitely no pretense. He introduced himself to me through kindness and, at times, humour, making the entire experience pleasurable. The hours passed in what seemed like minutes, and the memory of it has stayed in my mind as if it were yesterday; a truly special moment.

I waited until the following week before contacting Stephen Hurlbut, and we set up a meeting for the following day. A parking space was once again reserved for me and once again security escorted me to Stephen Hurlbut's office.

Shortly after checking in with his assistant, I caught the eye of a gentleman heading toward me. This must be Stephen, I thought.

"Hello Wendy and welcome. There's a quiet place just down the hall where we can talk."

I followed Stephen down and around the corridor until we arrived at a small room with a table and a few chairs. I introduced myself immediately.

"Hello Stephen," I said with my right hand extended. "I want to thank you for agreeing to meet with me."

I handed him a copy of my résumé along with a folder of press clippings like Jay Levine had passed on to Moses.

"I have had a discussion with Moses," Stephen said, "and he'd like to see something come of your work here in the newsroom. The pace in here is fast. We'll do what we can to help you gather a story, but I don't have a permanent place for you here right now. I've agreed to offer you a cameraman and have you go out and fetch a story for me."

"Gathering a story for you would be a great way to have you see my work, perhaps have something unfold eventually," I replied. "I'll be patient, Stephen."

I was grateful for the opportunity that I was being presented. I knew the television industry was incredibly competitive and therefore I was ready to jump at any possibilities open to me that would offer a more permanent television placement.

"I'll tell you what I can do," said Stephen. "You set the story up, get your subjects ready for the interview, and I will give you our seasoned cameraman, Jamie. Come back with your story, edit it, and you and I will talk."

"Yes, yes, I will definitely work on a story. What sort of time frame are we talking about?"

"You can give the Assignment desk a call in the morning. Let's see if we can set something up for later this week."

"I'll get to work on it right away," I replied.

I left 299 Queen Street West filled with optimism. Just what story I would set up became the ultimate question. I hoped to demonstrate not only my on-camera appeal, but my ability to seek out and secure story ideas that were worthy of the public's attention.

Chapter 21: Put to the Test

As I went through story ideas that evening, Lyndhurst Hospital came to my mind. This could be a practical piece to do, accessible to my physical limitations yet offering many different story angles. Even though it had been years since my stay there, I felt a story about Lyndhurst would be a chance to inform people about what was involved in rehabilitating someone who's sustained a spinal cord injury. I could also offer some insight into what I had been through myself.

I woke early the following morning knowing I had work to do. I began with a phone call to the Assignment Desk to secure Jamie, the cameraman Stephen Hurlbut had suggested the previous day.

"Assignment desk, John Thornton here."

"Good morning, John, this is Wendy Murphy. Stephen Hurlbut suggested I call you this morning to gain access to a camera before the week is up. Stephen said there was a cameraman by the name of Jamie that I'd be working with?"

"What day are you looking at, Wendy? I'll do my best to accommodate you," John replied.

"I'm aiming for this Friday morning, let's say around 10:00 a.m. Would that work for you, John?"

"Sounds great on my end, Wendy."

I hung up the phone only to be faced with new challenges: securing my interviews. While I had done numerous interview segments with YTV Canada, much of my work there was done by segment producers. Topics were chosen, those to be interviewed identified, and the segments ultimately edited by the producer in charge. In essence, my only job was to appear on camera, asking the questions that were often written by someone else. At City TV, it was now going to be up to me to pull my story together – from beginning to end.

I spent most of the day aligning my interviews for the coming Friday morning. I got in touch with the director of Lyndhurst, who would give me an overview of the facilities, and with a physiotherapist, who could provide some insight about what the patients admitted there now faced every day. Having this story unfold smoothly was paramount considering what was riding on the outcome. I'd been given the trust of both Moses Znaimer and Stephen Hurlbut to display my professional abilities, and I did not want to jeopardize that trust.

The night before my interviews, I ticked away like a time bomb to see my story completed. I was pleasantly surprised with a visit from my father. I loved our one-on-one time together. I always welcomed his words of wisdom; his perspective was a realistic reflection of the issues at hand.

"I'm not interrupting anything I hope," he said as he came through the door. "How was your day?"

"Very eventful," was my response.

My family was always very supportive of the endeavours I took on, but I wasn't sure I was prepared to let them all in on my project to become a professional television reporter. I didn't want them worried that the goal might prove too difficult to achieve.

"What's had you so busy?" he asked.

I decided I would confide in him.

"An opportunity of a lifetime has come to me, and I'm hoping things will work out. I've had meetings at City TV that appear promising. They've asked me to collect a story for them. I'm very excited at the prospect of getting hired there as a full-time reporter.

"That's great news, Wendy. Why so secretive?"

"I guess I was a little concerned that you would all feel I was reaching too high, career-wise. I know the television industry can be very competitive. I didn't want you to be worried about me. Maybe it's my own doubts that have kept me so quiet. Bottom line is I'll be doing a story for them tomorrow. I've already set up the interviews."

"That's incredibly exciting, Wendy. I am so happy for you. You know we love you as a family and that we always have your best interests at heart."

"Oh, I know that, Dad."

"And if things don't work out with City TV," my father added, "let's not forget all that you've already accomplished."

I knew he had a point. I had many achievements under my belt, some of which had seemed to fall right into my lap. Putting all the positive aspects of my life into better perspective was where my focus would stay.

"There's hardly a day that goes by when I don't think of Grania in one way or another, wondering where our friendship would be today. If it's not Grania, there are always the patients at Lyndhurst, the Angies and Steves, who have very limited use of their arms and hands. There are so many things I am very thankful for, not to worry there, Dad."

"Wendy, I don't want you to feel that we would discourage you as a family. Nothing could be further from the truth. Again, we want the best for you."

"You just wouldn't want me to set myself up for failure. I get it Dad, really."

"It's not failure that concerns me, just your overall expectations. It's important you don't lose sight of what you have already achieved," he added again, speaking in a caring tone of voice as he came over to offer me a hug.

Not long after our father-daughter talk, my dad said his goodbyes and headed out the door. He had chores to do, and it would never be his way to disappoint my mother.

The morning of my interviews arrived. For once there was no question as to where I was going or how I would get there: I definitely knew where Lyndhurst was located and that it was fully accessible. It had been years now since my discharge. It would be a surreal feeling, returning to a place that I had once relied upon to transform me, to gain a new form of independence. Without Lyndhurst I don't know how I would have adjusted to living life from the wheelchair; what the facility gave me was monumental in my recovery, not to mention all I learned from the patients I was blessed to have met there.

I made my way to the reception desk to have Randy Swan, the clinical director of Lyndhurst, informed that I had arrived. While I was waiting, I noticed a middle-aged man entering the hospital with a camera on his shoulder. I waved my arms in the air, making sure he saw me.

"Hi there, you must be Jamie." I asked. "I'm just gathering my contacts for the shoot. It shouldn't be long before we're ready."

Jamie went over to the lounge area to wait for us to get started, and soon Randy Swan appeared.

"Hello Wendy, pleasure to meet you."

"Hello Randy, and thanks for agreeing to the interview, I'm looking forward to it."

"Great! I also have a physiotherapist lined up for an interview. She works down around the gymnasium area, so we'll head that way when you are ready."

I wanted to have three individuals in my news segment, but time constraints were crucial. In the world of news programming, keeping stories informative yet concise is critical to programming. It is rare for a news story to run longer than two minutes in a one-hour newscast unless it's given priority as a lead story. The average air time per news segment falls around a minute and thirty seconds.

I now had Randy ready to take centre stage.

"Well Randy, there's no time like the present to get started. Let's have you stand over there by the double doors."

Randy and I made our way closer to the double doors and Jamie placed a microphone on the lapel of Randy's blazer.

"Check, check, 1, 2, 3...." I spoke into the hand-held microphone to ensure the frequency was clear for Jamie to hear.

"Now Randy, can we have you say your full name with spelling, and your formal title here at Lyndhurst Hospital?"

"R-A-N-D-Y-S-W-A-N, and my title is Senior Clinical Director."

With audio cleared by Jamie, I began with my questions.

"So tell me, Mr. Swan, what sets Lyndhurst Hospital apart from the many other rehabilitation facilities in the Toronto area?"

"That would be our knowledge of spinal cord recovery, Wendy. Patients here have made their way through the critical period they faced in the general hospital. They are now here to adjust to their new circumstances, with the most technological advances in the equipment and the expert staff we provide for someone living with spinal cord damage."

"Can you tell me a bit about the staff here?" I asked.

"We have nurses on all four hospital wings, with top-notch physio- and occupational therapists on hand to bring patients through the dynamics of regaining their physical independence. It's a process our staff takes pride in. No patient is discharged until that full range of independence has been achieved."

"And how long can patients expect to be here at Lyndhurst Hospital?"

"That would vary according to level of injury, but most are here anywhere from four weeks to four months."

"What are some of the real challenges patients here can expect to face, Randy?"

"It would be the process of adapting. Many come here with little knowledge of exactly what physical changes come when the spinal cord is compromised. Those with cervical lesions, or damage to the neck, would certainly have many challenges through this process."

"That's it Randy, you did well!" I assured him when we were finished.

After we wrapped things up, Randy directed me to where I would find the physiotherapist I would interview. Both Jamie and I followed the corridor around to the side of the hospital, where I was greeted by Beverley Bronson, a veteran physiotherapist at Lyndhurst.

I suggested that we do our interview in the gymnasium, since that was where most of the rehabilitation equipment was.

The full-circle aspect of it all hit me immediately after entering the gymnasium: this was a place where I had once spent months working out hard, all in preparation for life outside of rehabilitation. It had been years now, but somehow it felt like little time had passed. I was no longer jaded about what I could expect post-injury; I was determined, with a realistic view of what was now possible. I had found a new approach to life since my discharge, with a real purpose found while moving forward.

Putting all that was happening into perspective, I began with my questions.

"So tell me, Beverley, what role do you play in the recovery process of the patients here at Lyndhurst?"

"As a certified physiotherapist, my job begins with an assessment of the patient assigned to my care. We then put a physical routine into place for the duration of their stay here. I work in conjunction with doctors and perhaps the occupational therapist, if one is assigned. Our ultimate goal is to prepare the patient for eventual discharge."

"And what are some of the obstacles faced by these patients?"

"Well, I would not call them obstacles, but rather challenges. Patients here have sustained trauma to the spinal cord, and rehabilitation is crucial to bring them back into mainstream society. It takes hard work, and it is a continual challenge."

"In your opinion, Beverley, what is the greatest of those challenges?"

"Oh, Wendy, that's difficult to answer. I suppose it all begins with acceptance. While it may be a hard pill to swallow, coming to terms with the changes their body is facing, not to mention building the body's strength and endurance, is a crucial part of the overall recovery."

"That was great, Bev. Thank you so much for participating. Now, where might I find the patient who's agreed to take part in this story?"

"She's waiting for you in the reception area by the gymnasium. Her name is Chrystal Davids."

I knew exactly where to find her. It was where I had entered on my first day at Lyndhurst, while still on the ambulance stretcher. I remembered my first impression of the facilities and my initial excitement to finally be out of the general hospital.

When I got to the reception area, I introduced myself to Chrystal.

"I hope that I might have you come into the gymnasium for the interview. It provides some great visuals, with patients busy doing their workouts."

"But of course, Wendy, whatever will work for you."

I appreciated her flexibility. We all made our way back to the gym and I began my questions.

"I'm curious to know exactly what's brought you here to Lyndhurst, Chrystal."

"I was climbing a tree, and the branch let go. I fell at least eight feet and landed on my back."

"What diagnosis have they offered you? Is recovery possible at this stage?" I asked.

"A full recovery is likely," Chrystal said, while moving one leg straight out and back onto the foot plate of her wheelchair.

Wow, I thought. How lucky was she to have so much return. It was a quick thought before I moved on to my next question.

"What is a day in the life of Chrystal Davids like here in rehabilitation?"

"Well, with my full mobility expected to return, I've been exempted from the mat class they hold here for most newcomers. It's a class designed to prepare you for the full day of physio and often occupational therapies. Most of my workouts involve one-on-one sessions with my physiotherapist, or I work on weights and pulleys independently. It's been a real test of endurance."

"What have you learned through the entire experience?"

"Probably how quickly life can change. I was innocently tree climbing with my cousins when I took the fall; it was an activity we had done often with no serious consequences up until then. And I suppose I've learned about the resilience we can all show when faced with a difficult time."

"Well Chrystal, I can certainly relate to that. It was a motor vehicle accident that put me in a wheelchair, and we all drive in cars on a regular basis. You simply never know what life has in store for you, it seems. I want to thank you for your time and for your efforts in contributing to this story."

"Oh, it was no problem, Wendy. I'm happy I could help," Chrystal replied.

With the interviews complete, I ensured that Jamie had taken outside visuals of Lyndhurst Hospital, as well as interior shots to cover the story. I was confident that I had collected a good amount of material on the recovery process at Lyndhurst – certainly enough for a minute and a half of a finished news segment. I hoped it would illuminate the recovery process faced by those with spinal cord injuries.

Putting the actual story together would now be my next challenge.

***

A telephone call to the City TV newsroom set me up with an editor to help put together the story. While it is generally the reporter's job to put a story into proper context, a good editor can take a nothing story and really make it sing to an audience. I headed to the station immediately after completing Chrystal's interview.

"Hello Wendy, and welcome back," said Stephen Hurlbut when I arrived at City with my tape. "We have Dave Bourne here ready to work with you in the editing bay."

"That's great! I'm ready now if that will suit you."

Stephen was certainly following through with everything I needed to complete my story. I thanked him once more for his help.

It was not long before I was joined by Dave Bourne, who towered over me with his height.

"Hello Wendy, I understand you have a story in the can and ready to be edited."

"That's right, Dave, the interviews are all here. We just have to put them together."

I had paper-edited most of what I wanted. Betamax tapes include a feature that lets you edit using time code numbers. This allows for a more productive time while working in the editing bay with the assigned editor. When putting a story together, time constraints are first and foremost, all while trying to maintain the integrity of the story. Sound bites and visuals are a great way to break up the interviews, making the story more upbeat with a better flow while getting the message out to the viewer.

I began the story with a sound bite of a physiotherapist counting down from ten while a patient worked with weights. From there I went to a voiceover explaining the facilities in general and their capacity for full-time patients. I then moved on to Randy Swan, who described Lyndhurst as one of the few hospitals with advanced knowledge and expertise in treating patients dealing with traumatic spinal cord injuries. I introduced Chrystal after Randy, confirming her satisfaction with the facilities, before moving on to Beverley and her insights about treating patients at Lyndhurst Hospital. I finished the segment with what's called an extro, briefly stating the length of Chrystal's approximate stay and the number of patients estimated to seek treatment there that year.

"I want to thank you for assisting me with editing this story, Dave," I said when we were finished. "I think we put together a really compelling piece of work. My only question now is where I might find Stephen Hurlbut. He wanted to see the finished product."

"There's no mystery there, Wendy. Steve's office is in the far left corner of the newsroom."

Making my way over to Stephen's office, I experienced an array of emotions. On the one hand, I was finally closer to perhaps, acquiring a spot on television so that I could better represent the physically challenged community; on the other hand, my work might not live up to the expectations of Stephen Hurlbut and the standards set by City TV. I did not know what might come of the situation, but I was willing to accept whatever came my way.

I approached his office tentatively, knocking ever so lightly on the door.

"Come in, Wendy," he said.

"Well Stephen, I have fulfilled my end of the bargain. The story you requested is officially in the can. If you have some time now we could go over it together."

"By all means, I could make some time for you now, Wendy."

I approached Stephen with the demo tape in my right hand; passing it to him I added some humour to the moment.

"Here's your breaking news story for tonight's six o'clock news," I announced.

"Jokes aside, I am really looking forward to seeing what you've put together here, Wendy," he said, his words sounding sincere. "I'm always open to new story ideas."

We watched the tape together, and though I don't think it showed, I was busting with excitement. I could not believe what was happening. Here I was sitting in the VP of News Programming for City TV's office showcasing my work. It was like a dream; I was waiting to be pinched.

"It's a well-executed story, Wendy, very well done," said Stephen finally. "Unfortunately that doesn't change the fact that I have no job for you here at this time, not that that can't change in time. I like your work. It has potential to do well here, although I have nothing to offer you right now."

"Telling me that there's a good chance of gaining employment here is all I need to hear," I responded. "I would be honoured!"

***

As the old saying goes, good things come to those who wait. It was more than one year after the day I met with Stephen Hurlbut that I was actually hired as a contributing reporter for City TV. I was offered the segment I had asked Moses about during our meeting.

In September of 1995, I began Wendy's Video Diary, a feature of City TV weekend news that aired on the six o'clock and eleven o'clock newscasts for over eight years.

The video diary was a community-based concept covering a wide range of topics. Each segment ran on television for only a few minutes, but in that time I shared my own take on the world with the people who were watching.

In a way I felt I had come full circle in my journey from accident victim and hospital patient to full-fledged on-air professional, working at a major television station. I had at one time wondered how I was going to survive without the use of my legs while living in a world full of people who walked. Slowly, day by day, then month by month, and year by year, I set goals for myself and worked diligently to achieve them. I learned to become completely mobile in a wheelchair and to drive a car using just my hands; I became a model and a television actress; I skied down a mountain and even won a modelling contest. Throughout all of this, I was a spokesperson for the abilities – not the disabilities – of those using a wheelchair, and an advocate for public awareness of the external challenges we still sometimes face.

And now I was a television reporter bringing viewers into the lives of others who were reaching milestones: a celebrating centenarian or perhaps a couple acknowledging fifty years of marriage. I made my way into the homes of viewers. Some items were of a more serious nature such as stories of cancer survivors or organ recipients. I felt that this job was making use of all my abilities – those I had inside me and those I had learned along the way.

I roamed across the city of Toronto meeting people and bringing their heartwarming stories to life through my television camera and microphone. The idea of a person in a wheelchair being so mobile, travelling through the maze of our huge, often crowded city to seek and report human interest stories must have seemed revolutionary to some who saw Wendy's Video Diary. But it was an idea whose time, I thought, had definitely arrived. My thoughts were confirmed with the many awards I received while out in the field. My most rewarding acknowledgement came through Toronto Life Fashion Magazine when I was presented with the Woman Who Makes a Difference Award for the years I dedicated myself as a public figure. I was then inducted into the Who's Who of Canadian Women Directory, sharing the honour with a number of well-established Canadian women including the highly regarded television broadcaster, Pamela Wallin.

My job was not always an easy task. I often faced access challenges: venturing onto the uneven surfaces found in public parks, facing stairs at churches or community centres that still had no elevator or ramps, or simply being unable to get inside the homes of some of the guests that I interviewed. In every case I faced the challenge with an open mind, determined to overcome any barrier. I wanted my viewers to realize that those barriers were just temporary obstacles that could be overcome – that through effort, one day there could be a world without barriers.

Always in my mind was my mission to highlight the abilities of those of us who use a wheelchair but are not limited to what we can successfully contribute to society; we are limited not by our disabilities but by social attitudes. One we cannot change, but the other we definitely can – and continue to do.

Wendy Today

After spending more than three decades in a wheelchair, I have faced health issues in recent years, mainly some shoulder impairment due to overuse. Nothing, however, that has put my efforts to make a difference to complete rest.

After spending years hoping to mainstream the physically challenged community, today I focus my energies on access issues.

I am working on revisions to the accessible parking permit. This is the small blue-and-white placard-like sign with a wheelchair symbol clearly displayed that is usually placed on the dashboard or sun visor of any car transporting a person with a physical challenge. It enables holders of the permit to park in the disabled spaces that are made available at most public parking facilities. These designated spaces are larger than the average spots available to facilitate the wheelchair. Introduced in the late 80s/early 90s, these parking spaces are a vital component to my living independently while out in public.

Today it would seem there are simply too many permits in circulation, often authorized to those with walking ailments who are not necessarily in need of a wheelchair. The topic can be a sensitive one, sometimes challenging whose impairment is more worthy. I stand by my convictions that these spaces were initiated to facilitate a wheelchair. I was elated to see the program introduced and believe they should give those of us forced to use a wheelchair priority. We depend on the extra space offered in these designated spots to manoeuvre our wheelchairs in and out of our cars.

My efforts put forward to date have me working with Spinal Cord Injury (SCI) Ontario and March of Dimes Canada to revise the permit, while supporting the efforts of Gila Martow, MPP of Thornhill, Ontario. Ms. Martow has introduced a Private Member's Bill to the Ontario Legislature. Bill 39, Accessible Parking and Towing Industry Review Committee Act, 2018 requires the Minister of Government and Consumer Services to establish an advisory committee to do the following:

1.   Inquire into and report on the system of accessible parking for persons with a disability.
2.   Inquire into and report on matters related to the towing industry.

The committee is to be established within 90 days after the Bill receives Royal Assent and must report its recommendations to the Minister within eight months of its establishment. Within 60 days after receiving the committee's report, the Minister must then inform the Assembly of the recommendations that he or she will implement within the following five years.

The Bill is to establish a formal committee designated to review what currently does and does not work where the Accessible Parking Permit Program currently stands as a system.

When I'm not focusing my energies on accessibility, I am a peer support volunteer through SCI Ontario. With their office located right in the Lyndhurst Centre, peers are assigned according to age, sex, and level of injury. It is our hope as peer activists to prepare each patient for their ultimate discharge and the transition necessary in facing life outside of rehabilitation. It is a great concept that works well as a devised program, garnering public recognition for all of its positive results.

Printed in the USA
CPSIA information can be obtained
at www.ICGtesting.com
LVHW091917050924
790276LV00005B/106

9 781771 803465